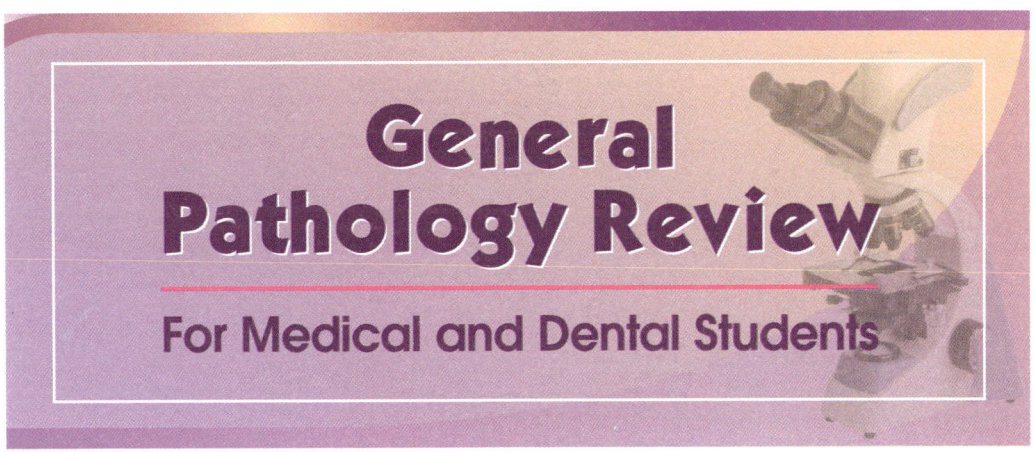

General Pathology Review

For Medical and Dental Students

SECOND EDITION

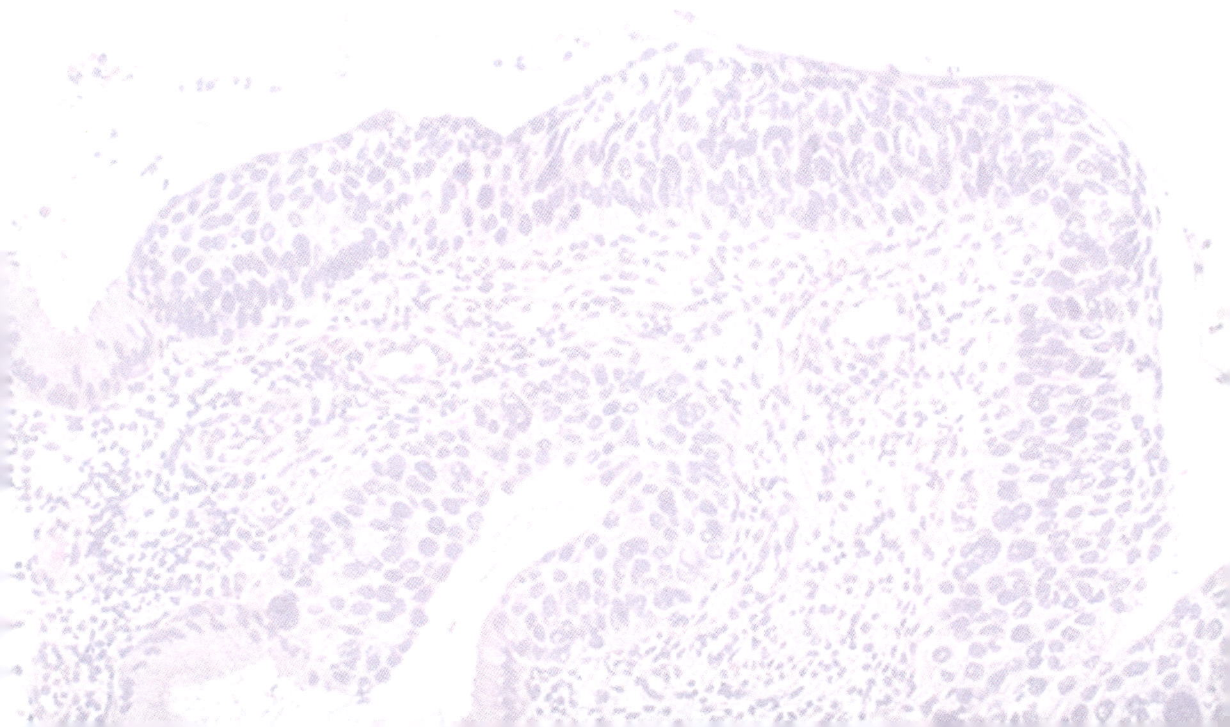

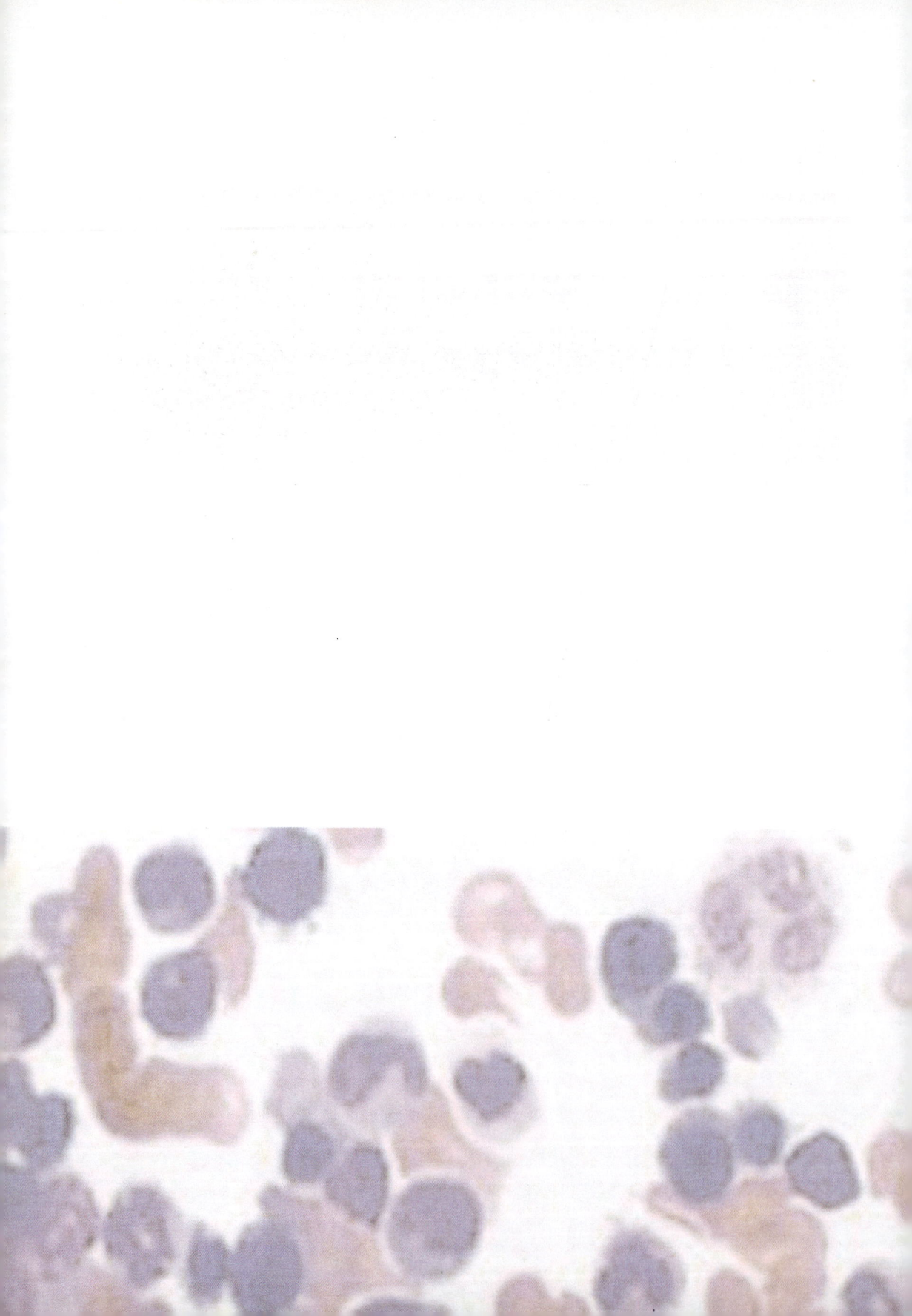

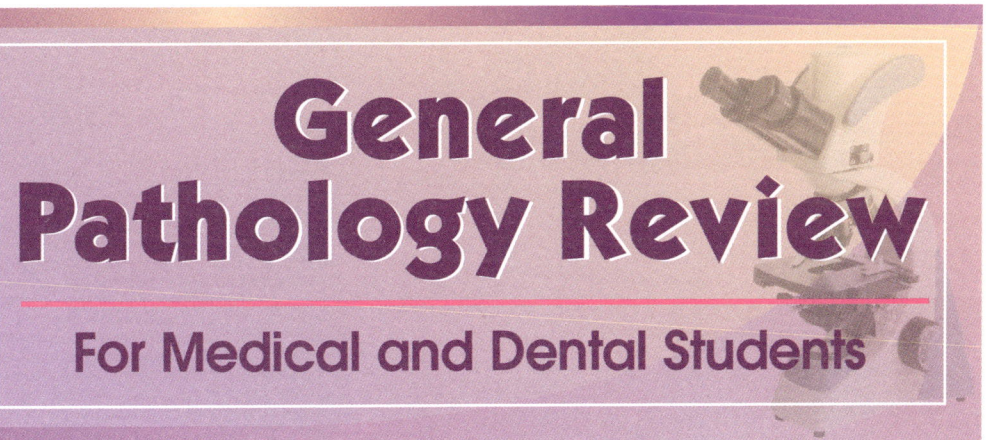

General Pathology Review

For Medical and Dental Students

SECOND EDITION

ML Gupta MBBS, MD (Pathology)

Associate Professor
Department of Pathology
Pacific Dental College
Debari, Udaipur (Rajasthan)

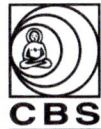

CBS

CBS Publishers & Distributors Pvt Ltd

New Delhi • Bengaluru • Pune • Kochi • Chennai
Mumbai • Kolkata • Hyderabad • Patna • Manipal

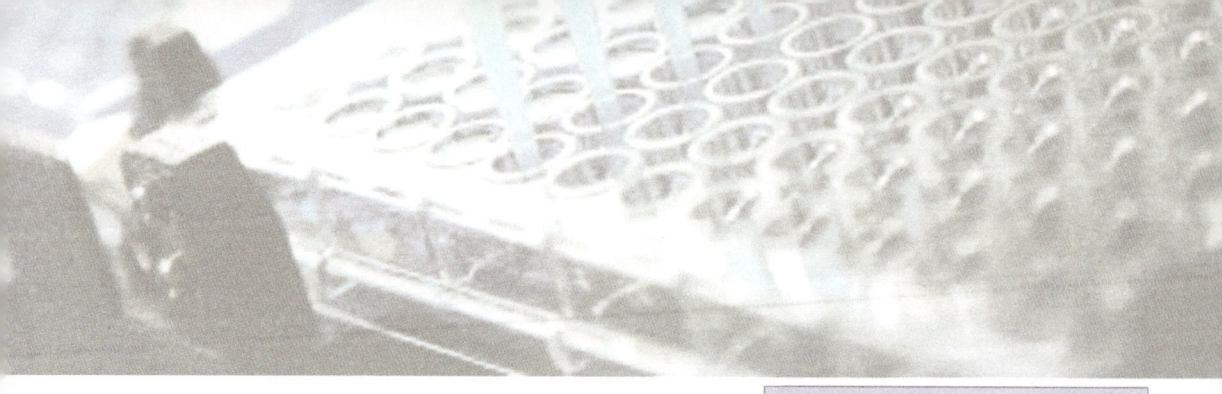

General Pathology Review

For Medical and Dental Students

Second Edition

ISBN: 978-81-239-2202-7

Second Edition: 2012
First Edition: 2009

Published by Satish Kumar Jain
CBS Publishers & Distributors Pvt Ltd
4819/XI Prahlad Street, 24 Ansari Road, Daryaganj, New Delhi 110 002, India.
Ph: 23289259, 23266861, 23266867   Fax: 011-23243014   Website: www.cbspd.com
e-mail: delhi@cbspd.com; cbspubs@airtelmail.in.
Corporate Office: 204 FIE, Industrial Area, Patparganj, Delhi 110 092
Ph: 4934 4934   Fax: 4934 4935   e-mail: publishing@cbspd.com; publicity@cbspd.com

Branches

- **Bengaluru:** Seema House 2975, 17th Cross, K.R. Road,
  Banasankari 2nd Stage, Bengaluru 560 070, Karnataka
  Ph: +91-80-26771678/79   Fax: +91-80-26771680   e-mail: bangalore@cbspd.com
- **Pune:** Bhuruk Prestige, Sr. No. 52/12/2+1+3/2 Narhe, Haveli
  (Near Katraj-Dehu Road Bypass), Pune 411 041, Maharashtra
  Ph: +91-20-64704058, 64704059, 32342277   Fax: +91-20-24300160   e-mail: pune@cbspd.com
- **Kochi:** 36/14 Kalluvilakam, Lissie Hospital Road, Kochi 682 018, Kerala
  Ph: +91-484-4059061-65   Fax: +91-484-4059065   e-mail: cochin@cbspd.com
- **Chennai:** 20, West Park Road, Shenoy Nagar, Chennai 600 030, Tamil Nadu
  Ph: +91-44-26260666, 26208620   Fax: +91-44-45530020   e-mail: chennai@cbspd.com

Representatives

- **Mumbai** 0-9833017933   • **Kolkata** 0-9831437309   • **Hyderabad** 0-9885175004
- **Patna**   0-9334159340   • **Manipal** 0-9742022075

Printed at Paras Offset Pvt. Ltd., C-176, Naraina Industrial Area Phase-I, New Delhi

Preface to the Second Edition

To study the alteration in cells due to disease at molecular level, resulting in morphological changes and presenting as symptoms, involves various specialities like molecular biology, cytology, biochemistry but it is the role of the pathologist to present a clear understanding and constitution of the disease.

General pathology includes cellular and structural alteration in the cell and host response involving interaction of haemodynamics. Study of general pathology is essential to understand the key concepts of illness for medical, dental and allied medical science students.

The basic aim of this book is to integrate and organize clear and concise concepts of pathological processes. After going through voluminous textbooks, students often get vague ideas about the subject but at the time of examination they are not able to recollect the facts. It has been an effort to arrange study material in digital and flowchart format. Emphasis has been given to the topics of clinical significance with adequate coverage and reasonable depth and details. Suitable illustrations and schematic diagrams will help the students in understanding the complicated interactions of pathological processes. Time tested organization of chapters has been followed to maintain the uniform approach.

I wish to acknowledge with gratitude the various authors of reference and textbooks which provided the authentic source material.

I wish to thank my wife Savita, my sons, my parents and all family members for their tolerance, unconditional support, affection, love and blessings. I am grateful to my esteemed teachers, my dear students, colleagues and friends for the various suggestions, their constant encouragement and moral support.

I avail this opportunity to thank CBS Publishers & Distributors Pvt Ltd for their efforts in bringing out this edition of the book in such an excellent form in four-colour format.

In spite of my best efforts, some errors might have escaped my attention and remained uncorrected in the text. I shall greatly appreciate for bringing up such errors to my notice. Suggestions are welcome for the improvement of the book.

ML Gupta

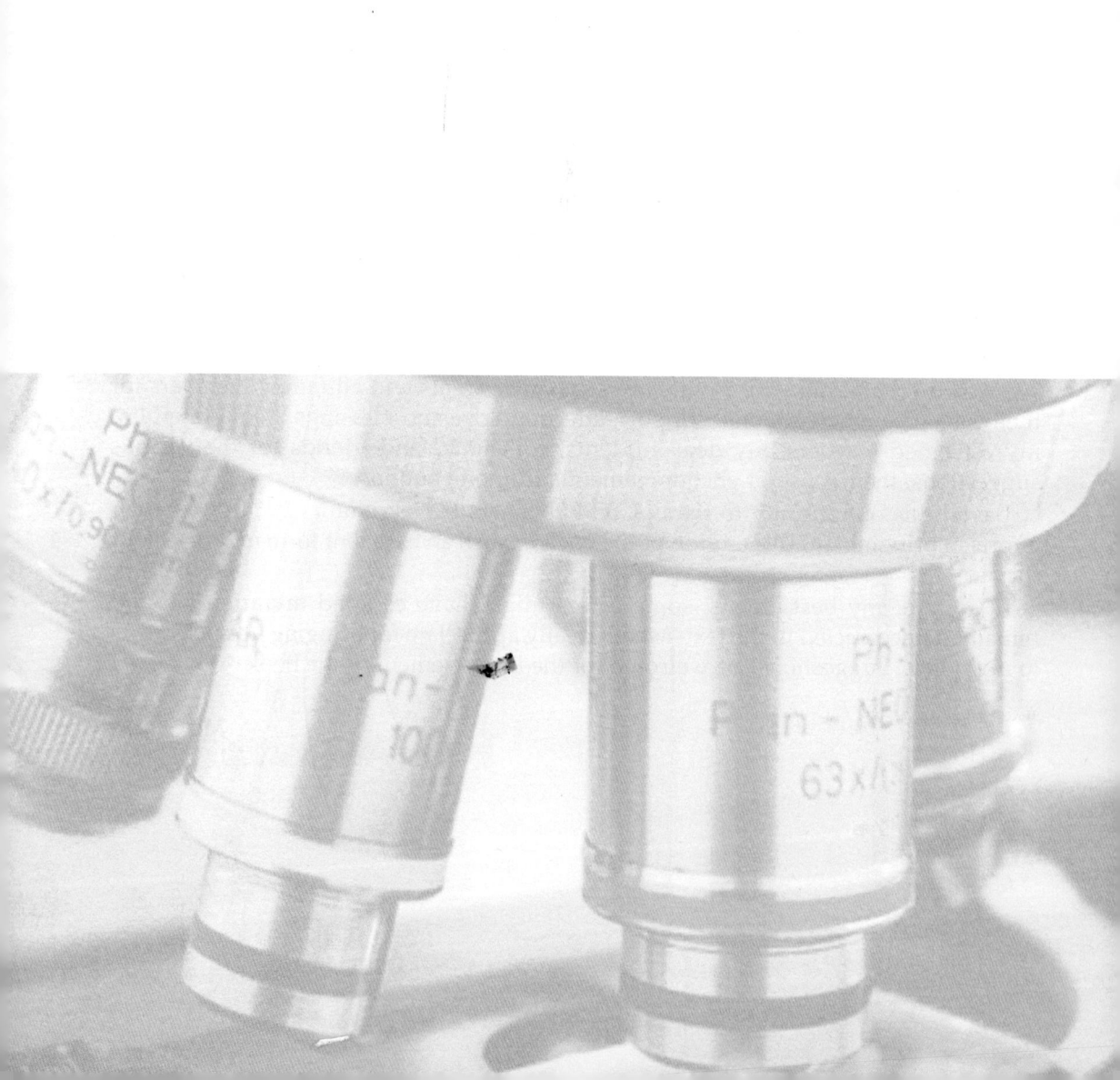

Contents

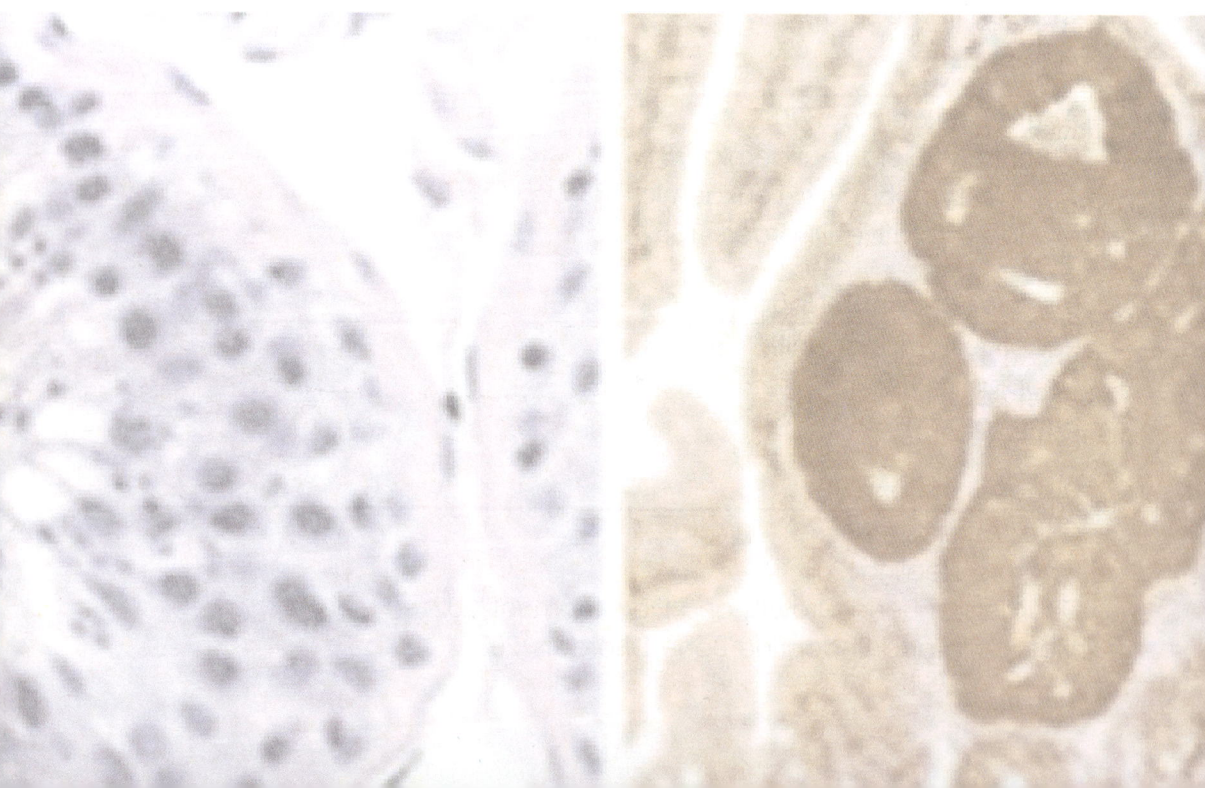

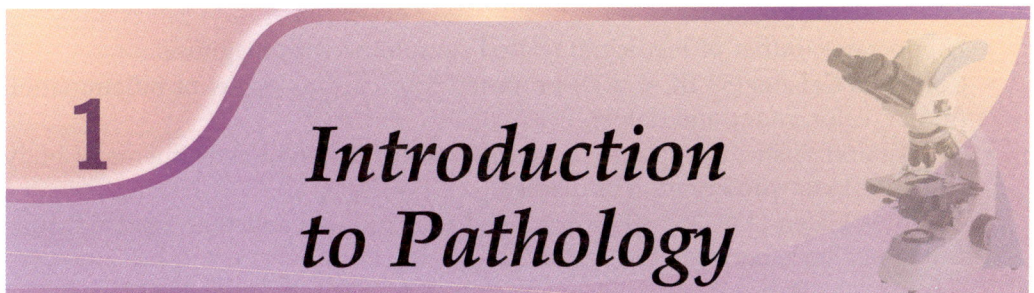

Introduction to Pathology

INTRODUCTION

Pathos: Suffering
Logos: Study

Pathology stands for "the study of suffering".
- It is the study of morphological changes in the cells, tissue, organ, organ system due to disease.
- From the clinical point of view, it is the branch of medical science:
  - To diagnose the disease,
  - To know the basic process of disease, and
  - To know the outcome of the disease, under the following heads.

1. Causation of disease (etiology).
2. Mechanism of development of disease (pathogenesis).
3. Structural changes in cells (morphology).
4. Functional consequences (clinical features).

Disease

Disease is defined in relation to health, as an alteration from the state of health.

Health is a state of well-being of
- Physical health
- Mental health
- Spiritual health

EVOLUTION OF PATHOLOGY

1. Supernatural belief—Initial concept about disease was that curse, evil eyes are responsible for the disease or illness.
2. Rational and philosophical approach—Socrates, Plato, Aristotle proposed concept of natural phenomenon about disease.

3. Logical approach (460–377 BC)
   - Hippocrates (father of medicine) related symptoms with diagnosis.
   - Cornelius Celsius (53 BC–7 AD) proposed four cardinal signs of inflammation (tumor, calor, rador and dalor).
   - Charka and Sushrut proposed disequilibrium of different constituents of body responsible for presentation of disease.
   - Claudius Galen (130–200 AD) postulated four humors and that disease results from imbalance between these humors.
4. Backward step. Rational approach was reversed during wide spread epidemics and death of people and again lead to supernatural concept that
   - Disease was defined as punishment for "sins".
   - Theory of vitalism (soul) emerged and belief was that disease results from hurting the soul and therefore dissection of human body was restricted.
5. Renaissance period. Study of anatomy and human body was started for the advancement of art and science, and dissection lead to discovery of various organs.
   - Leonardo da Vinci (1452–1519) painted human anatomy very precisely.
   - G Fallopius (1523–1562) discovered fallopian tubes.
   - GB Morgagni (1682–1771) established sequence of cause, lesion, symptoms and outcome of disease.
   - Sir Percivall Pott (1714–1788) identified cancer due to chimney soot and recognised it as carcinogenic agent (first occupational cancer).
   - John Hunter and William Hunter (1728–1793) established first pathologic anatomy museum.
   - Edward Jenner (1749–1823) invented smallpox vaccine.
   - Xavier Bichat (1771–1802) proposed that organ is composed of tissue and divided morbid anatomy into general and systemic pathology.
   - RTH Laënnec (1781–1826) described several lung diseases, chronic liver disease (Laënnec's cirrhosis) and invented stethoscope.
   - Karl F von Rokitansky (1804–1878) described acute yellow atrophy of liver, congenital heart defects and introduced concept of pathologist for diagnosis of disease.
   - Richard Bright (1789–1858) described non suppurative nephritis (Bright's disease).
   - Thomas Addison (1793–1860) described chronic adrenocortical insufficiency (Addison's disease).
   - Thomas Hodgkin (1798–1866) described chronic lymphoid disease, Hodgkin's disease.

a. Development of Cellular Pathology

   - van Leeuwenhoek invented microscope (1632–1723).
   - Marcello Malpighii studied capillaries, skin, spleen (father of histology).
   - Louis Pasteur assigned microorganism for causation of disease.
   - GHA Hansen isolated lepra bacilli as an etiologic agent of leprosy.

b. Development of Dyes and Stains to Stain Tissues

- Paul Ehrlich (1854–1915) developed Ehrlick's test for urobilinogen.
- Christian Gram (1853–1938) developed bacteriological staining by crystal violet (Gram stain).
- DL Romanowasky (1861–1921) developed eosin/methylene blue stain for peripheral blood film.
- Robert Koch (1843–1910) discovered tubercular bacilli and cholera organism, and described Koch's postulate and phenomenon.
- May Grunwald and Giemsa developed stain for blood and bone marrow cells.
- W Leishman (1865–1926) described Leishman stain for blood film and observed leishmania parasite as Leishman-Donovan bodies.
- Robert Feulgen (1884–1955) described Feulgen reaction in DNA and laid foundation of cytochemistry and histochemistry.

c. Development of Equipment and Machinery

- Rudolf Virchow (1821–1905) (father of modern pathology) developed histopathology as a method to study disease at cellular level.
- Cohnheim (1839–1884) introduced frozen section examination of tissue.
- Karl Landsteiner (1868–1943) invented blood group.
- Ruska and Lorries (1933) invented electron microscope.
- George Papanicolaou (1883–1962) developed exfoliative cytology.
- Tiju and Linen (1956) identified correct numbers of chromosomes in human.
- Watson and Crick (1953) proposed DNA structure.
- Nowell and Hagerford identified philadelphia chromosome in chronic myeloid leukaemia.
- William Boyed (1885–1958) a psychiatrist wrote book "Pathology for Surgeons".
- MM Wintrobe (1901–1986) discovered haematocrit technique.

Divisions of Pathology

1. Surgical pathology deals with study of tissue removed from living body.
2. Forensic pathology and autopsy deals with tissue removed at postmortem.
3. Cytopathology deals with the study of cells exfoliated or aspirated from body.
4. Hematology deals with the diseases of blood and blood forming cells.
5. Chemical pathology deals with biochemical analysis of blood and body fluids.
6. Immunology deals with immune system and immunological abnormalities.
7. Experimental pathology deals with study of diseases process in animals.
8. Geographic pathology deals with geographic disease distribution worldwide.
9. Medical genetics deals with relationship between disease and genes.
10. Molecular pathology deals with detection of abnormality in DNA at molecular level.

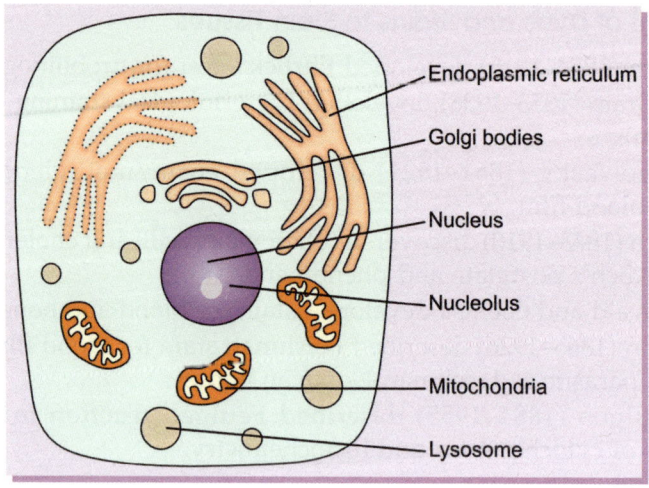

Fig. 1.1: Normal cell

The Normal Cell (Fig. 1.1)

1. Cell membrane
2. Nucleus
   - N. membrane
   - N. chromatin
   - Nucleolus
3. Cytosol and organelles
   a. Cytoskeleton
      - Microfilaments
      - Intermediate filaments
      - Microtubules
   b. Mitochondria
   c. Ribosome
   d. Endoplasmic reticulum (ER)
   e. Golgi apparatus
   f. Lysosomes
   g. Centrosomes
4. Intercellular junction
   - Occluding zone
   - Adhering zones
   - Desmosomes
   - Gap junction

2

Cell Injury

DEFINITION

The cell is exposed to external and/or internal stress. The response of the cell to injury/ stress depends upon the type of injurious agent and type of cells. As the result of injury following changes may take place

1. The cell may undergo morphological adaptive changes (cellular adaptations).
2. Post injury residual effect may persist, as
   - Subcellular changes or residual effect
   - Intracellular accumulation of normal/abnormal constituents/pigments (infiltration)
3. The cell may recover (resolution).
4. The cell may die (necrosis).

ETIOLOGY OF CELL INJURY

a. Genetic (Developmental, Karyotypic Defect, etc.)

Genetic injury leads to following defects
- Developmental defects like intrauterine death, growth retardation, malformation
- Cytogenetic defect—polyploidy, aneuploidy
- Simple gene defect—mutations
- Multifactorial inheritance disorders—cleft lip, diabetes mellitus, hypertension, congenital heart disease

b. Acquired

1. Hypoxia/ischemia/anemia
   - Due to lack of oxygen (hypoxia)
   - Due to decreased blood flow (ischemia)
   - Due to decreased oxygen carrying capacity (anemia)
2. Physical agents
   - Mechanical—Trauma, accidents
   - Thermal—Heat, burn

- Radiation—X-ray α-, β-, γ-rays
- Electricity—electric shock
3. Chemical
   - CN, carbon monoxide, As, Hg
   - Acid/alkali
   - Pollutants
   - Alcohol/drugs
4. Microbial
   Parasite/bacteria/virus/fungus
5. Immunological
   - Hypersensitivity reactions
   - Immune deficiency disease
   - Autoimmune disease
6. Nutritional
   - Deficiency diseases
   - Obesity, hypertension, atherosclerosis
7. Aging

Factors Affecting Consequences of Injury

- Type, duration and severity of agent: Small dose of toxic chemical for brief period of time induce reversible injury while large dose for longer duration may lead to death of the cell.
- Type, status, adaptability of target cell: Skeletal muscle can withstand hypoxia for longer duration without causing necrosis while myocardial muscle soon undergoes necrotic changes because of ischemia.

ISCHEMIC INJURY

Ischemia means lack of blood supply which leads to not only decreased oxygen and glucose supply but also increased accumulation of toxic metabolic products as the result of anaerobic ATP generation. Hypoxia means decreased oxygen content in the blood due to decrease or defective oxygen delivery to the tissue. Supply of glucose and removal of toxic metabolites is normal. Hence injury due to ischemia is faster and grievous than hypoxic injury.

Pathogenesis

With occlusion of end artery, for example coronary artery, up to certain extent injury is reversible but after that injury becomes irreversible. Time varies from tissue to tissue. In reversible injury if blood flow is restored some how, then paradoxically, the process of injury is further accelerated, known as reperfusion injury.

Biochemical Changes

- ATP depletion: Commonly it is seen in ischemic and toxic injury. In ischemic injury due to lack of blood supply, ATP production is decreased, since Krebs cycle requires oxygen for ATP production.
- Accumulation of byproducts: Lactic acid gets accumulated due to glycolysis. Oxygen derived free radicals get accumulated which are generated by mitochondrial respiration. Sequestrated calcium is released from mitochondria and endoplasmic reticulum. All result in deleterious cellular effect.

Metabolic Changes (Fig. 2.1)

- Oxidative phosphorylation and ATP production is decreased affecting membrane transport, protein synthesis lipid synthesis and phospholipid metabolism.
- Glycolysis is increased (anaerobic respiration) leading to production of lactic acid which lowers the pH of cytosol and causes clumping of nuclear chromatin.
- Protein synthesis is decreased due to detachment of ribosomes as the result of hypoxia affecting repair and cell growth.

Structural Changes

- *Cell membrane:* Decreased ATP leads to failure of sodium pump which regulates Na/K concentration in the cell.
- Cytoskeleton damage leads to distension of endoplasmic reticulum, swelling of mitochondria, appearance of blebs and loss of microvilli in cell membrane.
- *Nucleolus:* Decreased RNA and segregation of fibrillar and granular component is seen.

CHEMICAL INJURY

Chemical injury due to drugs, chemicals, and toxins induce sequence of events leading to cell death.

Pathogenesis

Direct injury: Chemicals and toxins directly combine with certain molecules or cell organelles inducing injury. For example, mercuric chloride binds to SH group of cell membrane and other proteins, leading to increased cellular permeability and inhibition of ATP dependent transport mechanism. Potassium cyanide blocks the oxidative phosphorylation when it combines with mitochondrial cytochrome oxidative enzymes.

Indirect injury: Certain substances are converted to reactive toxic products in liver and other tissues which cause lipid peroxidation by free radicals and form covalent bond with membrane proteins and lipids, for example carbon tetrachloride (CCl_4) is converted to CCl_3 and Cl^-. Free radical generated cause auto oxidation of fatty acid of phospholipids present in cell membrane.

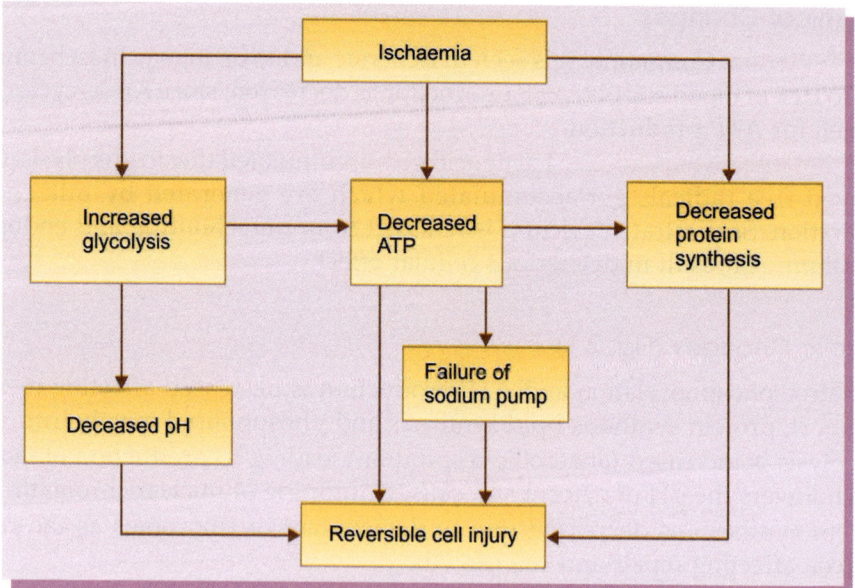

Fig. 2.1: Schematic diagram of reversible cell injury

PHYSICAL INJURY

Radiation: Radiation energy produce catastrophic biologic effects. Non-ionizing radiations produce vibration and rotation of atoms in biologic molecule, while ionizing radiation ionize biologic molecule and eject electrons.

Pathogenesis

Low doses radiation cause subcellular damage primarily to DNA. In high doses overt necrosis is seen. In intermediate doses proliferative cells are destroyed.

- DNA damage caused by particulate radiation, X-ray, γ-ray, or indirectly by oxygen derived free radicals induce activation of p53 which result in cell cycle arrest, DNA repair defect and apoptosis.
- Carcinogenic effect is produced due to genetic instability leading to delayed mutations accumulation. Persistence DNA damage which are not repaired is responsible for induction of cancers.
- Persistence of cytokines after initial exposure to radiation leads to fibrosis.

Mechanical

Mechanical force may inflict soft tissue, skin and bone in the form of abrasion, laceration, contusion, ulceration and fractures.

Thermal

Injury due to extremes of temperature especially burn is quite common. Depending upon extent and depth of burn severity of injury may vary. Prolong exposure to elevated temperature result in heat cramps, heat exhaustion and heat stroke. Hypothermia occurs due to prolong exposure to low ambient temperature. Freezing cells and tissues cause direct injury by crystallization of water. Indirect injury is produced by increasing blood viscosity.

Electrical

Electric current injury may vary from thermal injury to disruption of neural regulation.

Pressure Changes

High altitude illness is seen in mountaineers because of low oxygen tension. Compression wave from air explosion may collapse thorax or abdomen leading to rupture of internal organs. Decompression sickness is seen due to air or gas embolism.

MORPHOLOGICAL TYPES OF INJURY

A cell is born to perform its destined role till its lifespan. During its lifespan the cell is exposed to various external and internal pathological stimuli/stress, which affect the function of the cell. The cell undergoes various changes in the morphology in response to the external and internal injury or stress.

Following consequences may occur:
a. Reversible cell injury (retrogressive changes) (degeneration)
b. Residual effect (subcellular alterations)
c. Deranged metabolism (intracellular accumulation) (infiltrations)
d. Irreversible cell injury (necrosis)
e. Programmed cell death (apoptosis)
f. After effect of necrosis (gangrene, calcification)

Reversible Cell Injury (Cell Degeneration)

Types of reversible cell injury
1. Cellular swelling
2. Hyaline changes
3. Mucoid changes
4. Fatty changes

Cellular Swelling (Cloudy swelling, hydropic changes, vacuolar degeneration)

Increase in volume of cell because of accumulation of water is known as cellular swelling. It results from impaired sodium regulation due to failure of sodium pump. Sodium pump function depends upon ATP supply, therefore as the result of ischemia ATP production is decreased leading to cellular swelling. Solid organs like kidney, liver show earliest changes.

- *Gross features:* Kidney, liver, heart are enlarged and appear paler, more turgid and heavier.
- *Microscopic features:* Cells appear swollen, vasculature is compressed, and small clear vacuoles are seen in cytoplasm.
- *Ultrastructural features:* Endoplasmic reticulum appear distended, with detached polysomes, mitochondria appear swollen. Blebs are seen over the surface of cell membrane.

Hyaline Changes (Eosinophilic glassy appearance)

It is a kind of reversible injury in which pink material get accumulated inside the cell (intracellular) or outside the cell (extracellular). It is not specific substance but includes heterogeneous conditions.

Intracellular Hyaline

- Hyaline droplets are seen in tubular epithelium because of excessive reabsorption of plasma proteins in renal diseases.
- Hyaline degeneration (Zenker's degeneration) in typhoid fever—eosinophilic hyaline material is seen in skeletal muscle bundles.
- Mallory's hyaline body is seen in hepatocyte due to alcoholic liver cell injury.
- Hyaline inclusions are seen in various viral infections.
- Russell bodies seen in multiple myeloma are plasma cells (myeloma cells) distended due to excessive antibody production and accumulation inside the cell.

Extracellular Hyaline

- Hyaline degeneration in leiomyoma is pink material deposition outside the cell.
- Old scar become hyalinised and appear pink due to thick collagen bundles.
- Hyaline arteriosclerosis is condition when pink material is deposited in arterioles.
- Corpora amylacea is pink prostatic secretion in the lumen of prostatic glands.

Mucoid Changes (Mucin like material)

Mucoid means mucin like material. It is seen in reversible injury to epithelium leading to collection of mucoid material.

- Epithelial mucin is seen in inflammation of mucus membrane, mucocele, and mucus secreting tumors. Epithelial mucin gives positive reaction with PAS stain
- Connective tissue mucin does not give positive reaction with PAS stain. They are seen in mucoid degeneration, like myxoedema, ganglion wrist.

Fatty Changes

Certain cells which deal with fat metabolism when injured show intracellular deposition of fat in cytoplasm of cells pushing nucleus aside. It is called fatty changes or fatty degeneration. Usually liver, kidney and heart are affected.

Injury may occur due to:
- Excess alcohol consumption
- Saturation, malnutrition, chronic illness
- Obesity, diabetes mellitus
- Hypoxia
- Hepatotoxins (CCl_4, CH_3Cl, aflatoxin)
- Drugs (estrogen, steroids, tetracycline)

Mechanism of Accumulation of Fat (Fig. 2.2)

- Increase FFA mobilization due to starvation, toxins, diabetes mellitus, anoxia, obesity, alcohol

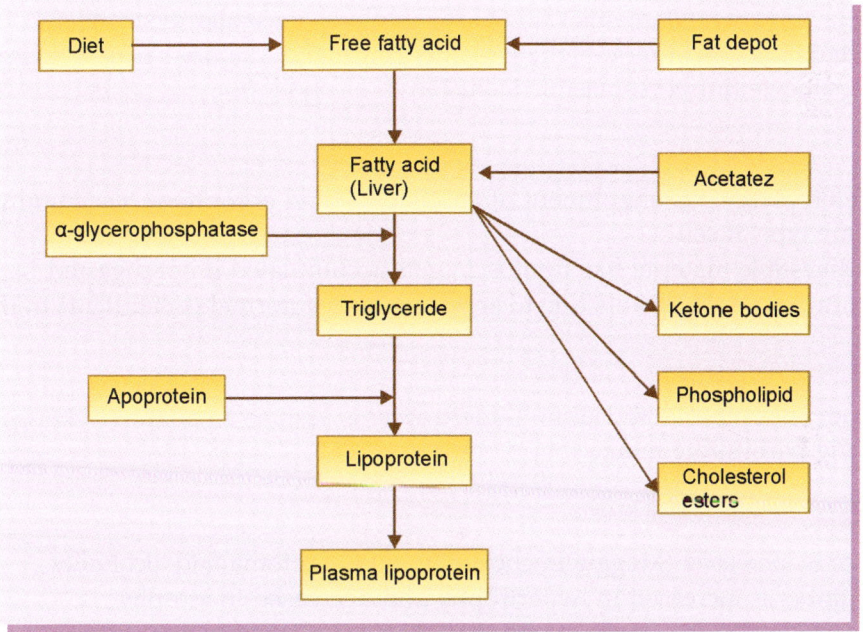

Fig. 2.2: Pathogenesis of fatty changes

- Increase fatty acid production by liver
- Decrease ketone bodies conversion of fatty acid due to anoxia, starvation
- Increase α-glycerophosphatase activity due to alcohol consumption leads to increased triglyceride in cell
- Decrease lipid acceleration protein due to CCl_4 toxicity, malnutrition
- Decrease lipoprotein excretion

Gross Features

Liver is enlarged with tense glistening capsule, cut section shows greasy, bulging surface.

Microscopic Features

- Fat vacuoles are seen in the cytoplasm
- Lipogranuloma may develop when lipid vacuoles get ruptured.

Residual Effect (Subcellular alterations)

Certain subcellular changes persist even after withdrawal of injurious agent. Such morphological changes and functional changes are seen in many conditions, for example:

1. Cytoskeletal Changes

- Defective microtubules leads to poor phagocytic activity of neutrophils (Chédiak-Higashi syndrome), poor sperm motility, immotile cilia syndrome
- Defective microfilaments leads to myopathies, muscular dystrophies
- Accumulations of intermediate filaments leads to Mallory's bodies formation in hepatocyte (intracytoplasmic inclusion in alcoholics)

2. Lysosomal Changes

- Heterophagy, i.e. engulfment of another cell and autophagy, i.e. engulfment of same type of cell
- Indigestible material like lipofuscin gets accumulated if not digested
- Storage diseases results due to accumulation of normal constituents in the cell

3. Smooth Endoplasmic Reticulum

Smooth endoplasmic reticulum hypertrophy is seen as an adaptive change due to prolong barbiturate intake.

4. Mitochondrial Changes

- Size is increased (Mega mitochondria) in oncocytoma and alcoholics
- Number is increased in hypertrophy and decreased in atrophy

Deranged Metabolism (Infiltration or intracellular accumulation)

Injuries which derange metabolic function results into accumulation of certain substances inside the cell. It is known as infiltration of intracellular accumulation.

a. Accumulation of normal constituents inside the cell which are produced by normal metabolism like fat, protein and carbohydrate, for example, steatosis or fatty changes in liver.

b. Accumulations of abnormal substances inside the cell produced by abnormal metabolism leads to various storage diseases. For example, glycogen is accumulated in macrophages in Gaucher's disease (glycogenoses).

c. Accumulation of pigments like melanin and hemosiderin in many diseases like melanoma and hemosiderosis (Fig. 2.3).

Intracellular Accumulation of Fat

- Fatty changes (see in fatty changes)
- Cholesterol infiltration is seen in hypercholesterolemia which results in fibro fatty plaque formation in atherosclerosis. Presence of lipid vacuoles in the cytoplasm of histiocytes leads to formation of foam cell which is seen in xanthoma.

Intracellular Accumulation of Protein

- Excess of protein which is filtered through glomerulus is reabsorbed by proximal tubular epithelium and form hyaline droplets in the cytoplasm.
- Russell body formation is excessive accumulation of immunoglobulin in plasma cells which is seen in multiple myeloma.
- In α-1 AT deficiency, eosinophilic deposit of mutant protein is seen in cytoplasm of hepatocytes.
- Mallory's body accumulation is seen in hepatocytes in alcoholics.

Intracellular Accumulations of Glycogen

- In diabetes mellitus, high plasma level of glucose leads to accumulation of glycogen in the cells.
- Glycogenoses is a genetic disease in which deranged glycogen metabolism leads to accumulation of glycogen.

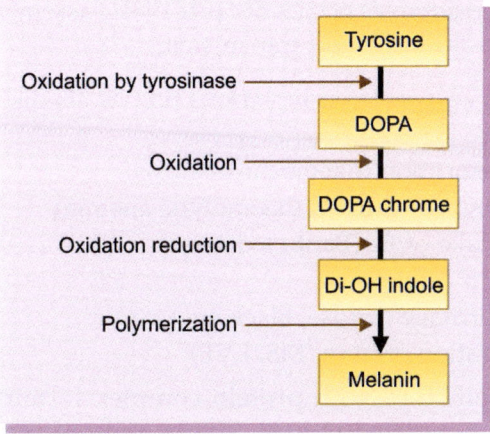

Fig. 2.3: Melanin synthesis

Intracellular Accumulation of Pigments

Pigments accumulated in the cells may be derived from endogenous sources, for example, melanin, homogentisic acid, haem derived pigments or lipofuscin. Pigments may be inhaled, ingested or inoculated from exogenous sources, for example, coal dust, silica and iron asbestos.

Endogenous Pigment Accumulation

a. *Melanin:* It is synthesized by melanocytes and dendritic cells by following process. Excess of melanin pigment is known as hyperpigmentation.

Hyperpigmentation is seen in following conditions:
Generalized: Addison's disease, chloasma (seen in pregnancy), arsenic poisoning.
Local: Neurofibromatosis, melanosis coli, lentigo.

Hypopigmentation: Decreased pigmentation is seen in following conditions:
Generalized: Albinism (tyrosinase actively in defective)
Localized: Leukoderma, vitiligo, leprosy, healing, DLE.

b. *Homogentisic acid:* Ochronosis is dark coloration of fibro cartilaginous tissue and urine due to accumulation of homogentisic acid. It is an autosomal recessive defect which manifest as deficiency of oxidase enzyme, required to break homogentisic acid. Homogentisic acid is excreted in urine. Urine becomes dark on standing the condition is known as alkaptonuria.

c. *Haem protein derived pigment:* Various haem derived pigments are hemosiderin, haematin, bilirubin and porphyrin

1. *Hemosiderin:* Iron and apoferritin combine to form ferritin. It is phagocytosed by macrophages and converted into haemosiderin. Excessive accumulation of haemosiderin is called hemosiderosis. It is of two types:
   a. Primary hemosiderosis occurs due to unknown cause (idiopathic).
   b. Secondary hemosiderosis occurs because of thalassemia, sideroblastic anemia, alcoholic cirrhosis, and blood transfusion.

   Hemosiderin gets accumulated in various tissues. Its distribution may be:
   - Generalized due to
     - Excess Fe absorption (haemochromatosis)
     - Excessive RBC breakdown (haemolytic anemia)
     - Excessive intake of Fe (Bantu's disease)
   - Localized due to
     - Local haemorrhage (bruise, black eye)
     - Brown induration of lung (MS, LVF)

2. *Haematin:* Iron combines with protein complex forming haematin pigment. Haematin gets accumulated in liver, spleen and reticuloendothelial tissue. For example, in chronic malaria and mismatched blood transfusion reactions.

3. *Bilirubin:* Porphyrin derived from break down of RBC is converted into bilirubin and conjugated in liver to be excreted in bile. Accumulation of yellow pigment (bilirubin) is seen in:
   a. Prehepatic jaundice (haemolytic anemia)
   b. Hepatic jaundice (hepatic disorders)
   c. Posthepatic jaundice (obstruction in bile duct)

4. *Porphyrin:* Tetrapyrrol ring combines with iron to form haem. Genetic deficiency of enzyme which is required for this reaction leads to excess of porphyrin left over. Accumulation of porphyrin is called porphyria. It is of two types:
   i. Erythropoietic porphyria (when defective haem synthesis occurs in RBC)
      • Congenital uroporphyria (urine appear red)
      • Erythropoietic protoporphyria (no red urine)
   ii. Hepatic porphyria (when defective haem synthesis occurs in liver)
      • Acute intermittent porphyria
      • Variegated form (seen in South Africa)
      • Hereditary type (rare)
      • Porphyria cutanean tarda

d. *Lipofuscin (Fuscus means brown):* It is brown lipid-protein complex derived from old atrophied cells, which is not digested by macrophages form wear and tear residual body. Accumulation of such pigment imparts brown discoloration to the organ. For example:
   • Brown atrophy of myocardium
   • Senile dementia (brown pigment in neurons)
   • Yellow brown granular material in hepatocytes and Leydig cells of testis.

Exogenous Pigment Accumulation

1. Inhaled
   • Carbon/coal dust accumulated in lungs lead to anthrocosis
   • Silica/stone dust accumulated in lungs lead to silicosis
   • Iron and iron oxide
   • Asbestos accumulated in lungs lead to asbestosis
2. Ingested
   • Silver salt accumulation in tissue is called argyria
   • Lead poisoning leads to blue lines over teeth
   • Carotenaemia is excess carotene in blood due to carrot taken in excess
3. Inoculations into the skin (tattooing)
   • India ink imparts black color
   • Cinnabar is used for red color tattooing

Irreversible Cell Injury (Cell death)

It is characterized by structural and functional changes which do not revert back to normal even after removal of injurious agent, i.e. cell death.

Intracellular Changes Observed in Cell Death

1. Mitochondrial dysfunction
   Vacuoles and calcium salt deposition is seen in mitochondrial matrix because of influx of Ca^{++}

2. Membrane damage is brought about by
   - Accelerated degradation of membrane phospholipids by activation of endogenous phospholipases
   - Cytoskeletal damage and hydropic changes by intracellular proteases
   - Free radical (O_2^-, OH^-, H_2O_2) attacks on polyunsaturated fatty acid (PUFA) of membrane called lipid peroxidation
3. Lysosomal membrane damage leads to liberation of hydrolytic enzymes, which cause digestion of cellular components

Types of Cell Death

1. Autolysis (self digestion)
2. Necrosis (death by injurious agents)
3. Apoptosis (programmed death)

1. Autolysis (Self digestion)

Autolysis is disintegration of cell by its own lysosomal hydrolytic enzymes. When cell death occurs due to enzymes derived from immigrant neutrophils, the process is called heterolysis. When occurs in living body, it is surrounded by inflammatory cells. When occurs in dead body it is not accompanied by inflammation. Rapid autolysis is seen in pancreas, gastric mucosa which is rich in hydrolytic enzymes. Fibrous tissue undergoes slow autolysis. Heart, liver and kidney show intermediate speed of autolysis.

Morphological Features

Tissue shows eosinophilic homogeneous cytoplasm with loss of cellular details and degradation of nucleus.

2. Necrosis

Necrosis is defined as focal death and degradations of tissue by hydrolytic enzymes accompanied by inflammatory reactions. Presence of inflammation signifies cell death in living tissue.

Morphological Features

Cytoplasm appear homogeneous eosinophilic because of
- Loss of basophilia which is imparted by RNA and
- Denaturation of intracytoplasmic proteins

Nucleus Shows (Fig. 2.4)

- Pyknosis (shrinkage of nuclear chromatin material)
- Karyolysis (dissolution of chromatin material)
- Karyorrhexis (fragmentation of nuclear chromatin material)

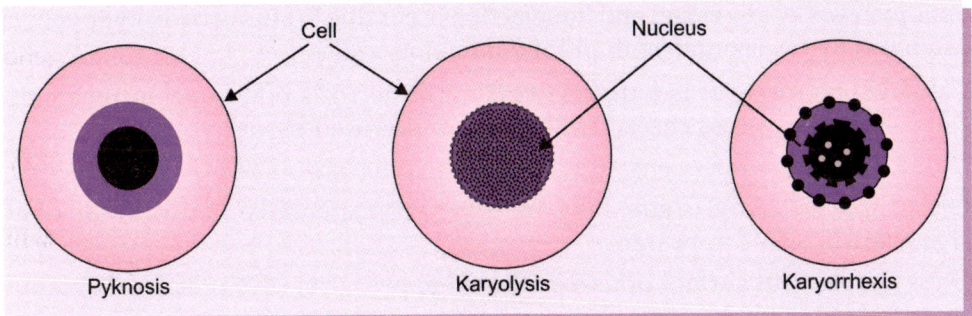

Fig. 2.4: Nuclear changes in necrosis

Types of Necrosis (Fig. 2.5)

a. Coagulative necrosis—It is characterized by death of the cell with preservation of cellular outline due to coagulation of cell proteins.

Causes: Ischemia, bacterial and chemical agents.

Organ affected: All organs except brain show coagulative necrosis like heart, kidney, and spleen.

Gross features: Organ appear pale, yellow, soft to firm, swollen or shrunken.

Microscopic features
• Cellular outline is well preserved
• Cytoplasmic and nuclear details are lost
• Inflammatory cell infiltrate is present with phagocytosis of cellular debris

Basic process: Cell structural proteins as well as enzyme proteins all undergo denaturation so that proteolysis process does not take place in the absence of enzymes and hence cell outline is preserved. Dead cells are later phagocytosed and digested.

b. Liquefactive necrosis—It is a type of necrosis characterized by formation of liquid viscid mass (pus) with accumulation of inflammatory cells.

Causes
• Ischemia, bacterial and fungal infections evoke marked inflammation so that necrosed tissue is transformed into pus
• In brain tissue hypoxia causes liquefactive necrosis

Organ affected: Brain and abscess cavity in any organ.

Gross features: Soft tissue with liquified centre filled with pale yellow viscid necrotic debris is known as abscess.

Microscopic features
• Necrotic debris and macrophages with phagocytosed material are seen
• Proliferating capillaries, inflammatory cells and glial/fibroblasts surrounds the liquified material

Basic process: Cell digestion and liquefaction occur due to strong hydrolytic enzymes produced by microorganisms and inflammatory cells.

c. Caseative necrosis—It is a distinctive kind of necrosis often seen in tuberculosis characterized by gross cheesy appearance of necrosed tissue

Cause: Tubercular infections

Organ affected: Any organ may be affected; especially lymph nodes show characteristic gross appearance.

Gross features: Cut surface of tissue affected appear dry, cheese like, soft, granular.

Microscopic features: Amorphous, eosinophilic, granular cellular debris surrounded by modified macrophages (epithelioid cells) wall off from surrounding tissue by fibroblast, lymphocytic infiltrate along with characteristic Langhans' type giant cells. This kind of focal lesion is known as granulomatous lesion.

Basic process: Coagulative and liquefactive necrosis occur simultaneously due to lipopolysaccharide present in the capsule of tubercular bacilli, which evoke delayed hypersensitivity reaction.

d. Fat necrosis—It is characterized by focal area of fat destruction in pancreas and peritoneal cavity by lipase enzyme.

Causes: Trauma, infection affecting pancreas

Organs affected: Pancreas, breast adipose tissue

Gross features: Firm deposits of chalky white calcium soap like material is seen on the surface of adipose tissue

Microscopic features
• Cloudy fat cells are seen with amorphous granular basophilic material
• Inflammatory cells are seen in the vicinity

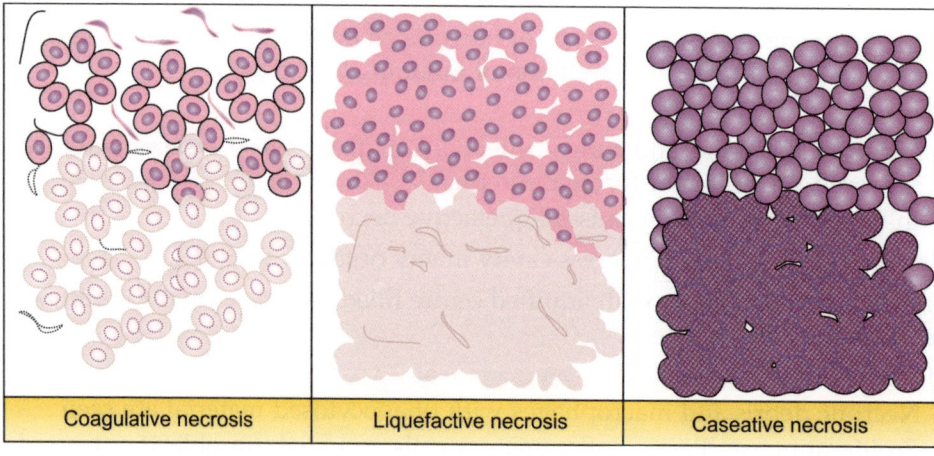

| Coagulative necrosis | Liquefactive necrosis | Caseative necrosis |

Fig. 2.5: Types of necrosis

Basic process: Pancreatic lipase enzyme cause hydrolysis of neutral fat, and split it in to glycerol and free fatty acid. Free fatty acid when combine with Ca^{++} calcium soap is formed. This process is known as saponification.

E. Fibrinoid necrosis—It is characterized by collection of fibrin like material at the site of necrosis.

Causes
- Immunologic tissue injury like vasculitis, autoimmune disease, Arthus reaction
- Hypertension
- Peptic ulcer

Organs affected: Blood vessels are predominantly affected

Gross features
- Fibrin like material is deposited in vessel wall
- Haemorrhage may occur due to rupture of blood vessel

Microscopic features
- Bright eosinophilic hyaline like material is observed in vessel wall
- Haemorrhage is seen where vessel ruptures

Basic process: Immunological reactions lead to destruction of tissue along with activation of coagulation cascade leading to precipitation of fibrinoid material.

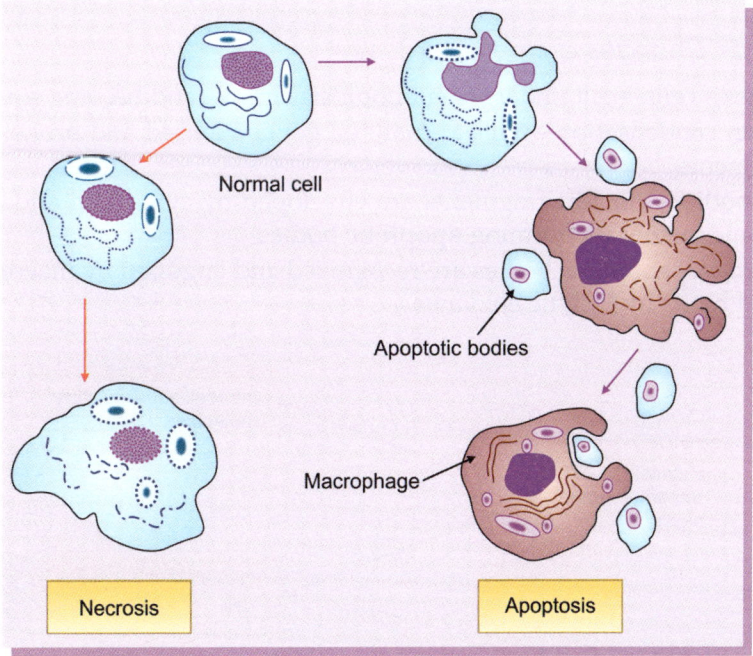

Fig. 2.6: Process of necrosis and apoptosis

3. Apoptosis

Apoptosis means "Falling off or Dropping off". It is defined as coordinated internally programmed death of cell or tissue. It is physiological as well as pathological condition.

Etiology

Programmed cell death is observed during conditions
• Development
• Homeostasis
• Defense mechanism
• Aging process

Physiological events
• Embryogenesis and foetal development
• Menstrual cycle (hormone dependent)
• Proliferating cells (epithelial cells)
• Neutrophil and immature T&B cell death

Pathologic conditions
• Cell death during tumor growth
• Atrophy of organ after duct obstruction
• In viral disease, damaged cells deletion
• Low dose injury by heat, radiation and drugs

Morphologic Changes during Apoptosis

• Shrinkage of cells—cell undergoing apoptosis shrinks and become smaller
• Chromatin condensation—nuclear material get condensed and broken into many tiny fragments
• Apoptic bodies—nuclear fragments are enveloped by cytoplasm and enclosed by cytoplasmic membrane forming apoptotic bodies
• Phagocytosis—apoptotic bodies are recognized and engulfed by macrophages and destroyed by its hydrolytic enzymes

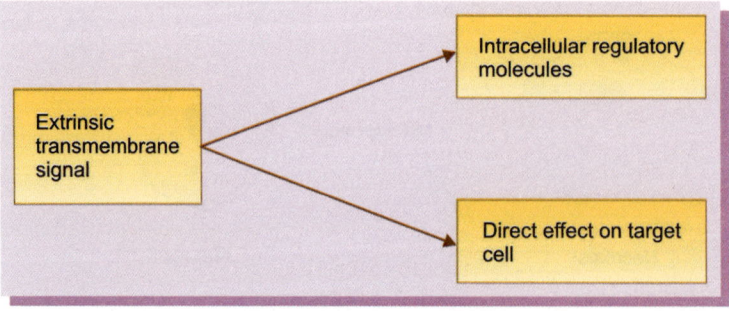

Fig. 2.7: Extrinsic pathway

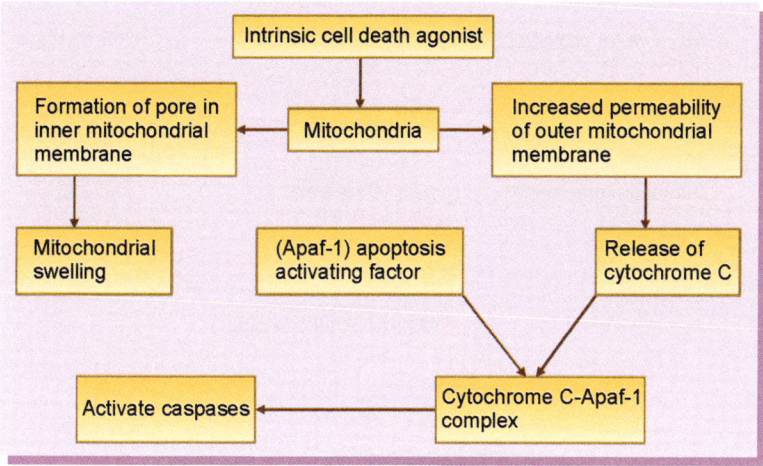

Fig. 2.8: Intrinsic pathway

Biochemical Changes

- Proteolysis of cytoskeletal proteins
- Protein-protein cross linking
- Fragmentations of nuclear chromatin by activation of nuclease
- Appearance of phosphotidyl serine on outer surface of cell membrane. In some forms thrombospondin appears over surface
- Early recognition by macrophages for phagocytosis

Mechanism of Apoptosis

a. Initiation of apoptosis (signaling)

Extrinsic pathway
- Negative stimuli (absence of growth factor cytokines, hormones required for normal cell survival).
- Positive stimuli (receptors for TNF)
- Intracellular stimuli (heat, radiation)

Intrinsic pathway
- Death agonists damage mitochondria leading to release of cytochrome C in cytosol
- Cytochrome C and Apaf-1 activates caspases

b. Regulation of apoptosis

Apoptosis is regulated by bcl-2 family of proteins
- Proteins located in mitochondrial membrane
  - Proteins bind to *bax* and *bad* proteins to promote apoptosis
  - Proteins bind to *bcl-XL* protein to inhibit apoptosis

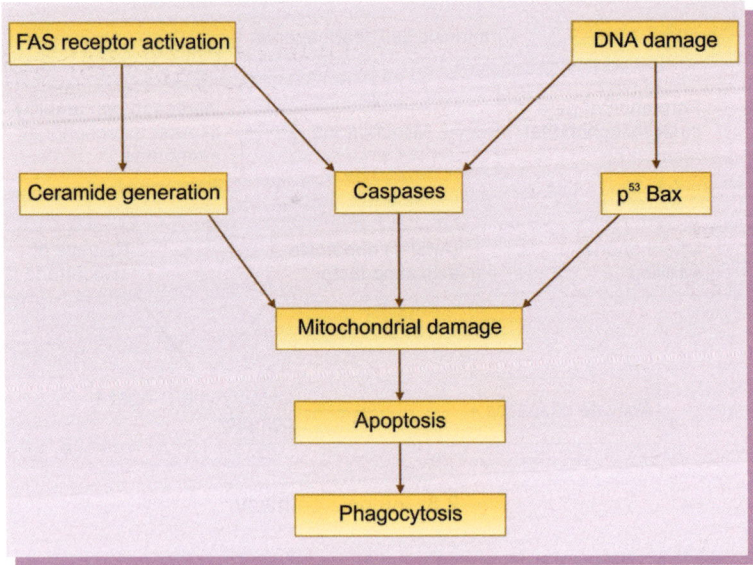

Fig. 2.9: Execution of apoptosis

- Proteins located in cytosol
  Pro-Apaf-1 (Pro-apoptotic protease activating factor) promote apoptosis
- c. Execution of apoptosis
  1. FAS receptor activations
     - FAS (CD 95) present on cytotoxic T cells, on coming in contact with target cells, are activated leading to activations of caspases and subsequently proteolysis.
  2. Ceramide generation: Syringomyelin of plasma membrane undergo hydrolysis with ceramide generation, which cause mitochondrial injury
  3. DNA damage: Ionizing radiations cause DNA damage (damage nuclear protein p^{53}) which induce cell death promoting protein (*bax*)
- d. *Phagocytosis, without inflammation:* Apoptotic bodies possess cell surface receptors which facilitates identification by phagocytic cells.

Difference between necrosis and apoptosis

Features	Necrosis	Apoptosis
1. Cause	Hypoxia, toxins, physical, chemical, microbial, immunological	Physiological and pathological conditions
2. Histology	Cellular swelling, disruption of nucleus and organelles	Shrinkage of cell, chromatin condensation and apoptotic bodies formation

Contd...

Contd...

Features	Necrosis	Apoptosis
3. Process	Random and diffuse nuclear changes, ATP depletion, membrane injury	Internucleosomal gene activation of endonucleases and proteases
4. Tissue reaction	Inflammation and phagocytosis	Phagocytosis without inflammation

GANGRENE

Definition

Necrosis superadded with putrefactions is known as gangrene.

Basic Process

Coagulative necrosis undergoes liquefaction by putrifying bacteria.

Classification

a. Dry gangrene
b. Wet gangrene
c. Gas gangrene

1. Dry Gangrene

Causes

Ischaemia in distal part of limb caused by arterial occlusion in the following diseases
- Atherosclerosis
- Thromboangiitis obliterans (TAO or Burger's disease)
- Raynaud's disease
- Ergot poisoning

Morphological Features

- Affected part appears dry, shrunken and black
- It spreads upwards, forming line of demarcation between gangrenous and healthy area
- Black color is due to iron sulfide formed by reaction of hydrogen sulfide on iron present in haem. Hydrogen sulfide is produced by bacteria
- Inflammatory granulation tissue is seen at line of demarcation

Prognosis

Better than wet and gas gangrene, with little septicemia

2. Wet Gangrene

Cause

Commonly venous obstruction, less often arterial occlusion in
- Moist tissue and organs (bowel, lungs, cervix, vulva, etc.)
- Diabetic foot (high plasma sugar level)
- Bedsores (bedridden patients)

Morphological Features

- It spreads to whole organ and septicemia develops due to toxins derived from bacteria
- There is no line of demarcation between affected and healthy area
- Affected part appears soft, swollen and putrid

Prognosis

Intense inflammation and numerous bacteria, leading to septicemia makes prognosis poor

3. Gas Gangrene

Cause

Wound contaminated with Clostridia, gas forming bacteria (gram-positive anaerobic bacilli) results in gas gangrene

Morphological Features

- Toxins released from bacteria cause necrosis and edema. Toxins absorbed systematically leads to septicemia
- Part affected appear swollen, edematous, dark brown and crepitant
- Wound appears foul smelling due to hydrogen sulfide produced by bacteria.

PATHOLOGIC CALCIFICATION

Definition

Deposition of calcium salt at sites other than osteoid or enamel is known as pathological calcification.

Types

1. *Dystrophic calcification:* It is deposition of calcium in dead or degenerated tissue with normal calcium metabolism and, calcium level in plasma.
   - Dystrophic calcification in dead tissue occurs: In caseative necrosis, liquefaction necrosis, fat necrosis, infarction, thrombus haematoma, parasites, breast cancer, etc.

- Dystrophic calcification in degenerated tissue occurs: In old scars, Mönckeberg's sclerosis, stroma of tumors, psammoma bodies, epidermal cyst, calcinosis cutis, senile degenerative changes
2. *Metastatic calcification:* It is deposition of calcium in normal tissue because of deranged calcium metabolism, and hypercalcaemia. Deposition occurs in blood vessels, kidney, lung and gastric mucosa.

Morphological Features

Deeply basophilic, irregular, granular material is seen in intercellular/extracellular or both locations.

Pathogenesis

Dystrophic Calcification

Local alteration of pH and release of enzymes (alkaline phosphatase) favors deposition of calcium.

Metastatic Calcification

Hypercalcaemia is responsible for calcium deposition. Hypercalcemia is due to excessive mobilization of calcium from bones and excessive absorptions from gut.

- Causes of excess mobilization
  - Hyperparathyroidism
  - Bone destructive lesions
  - Multiple myeloma
  - Metastatic carcinoma
  - Prolonged immobilization
- Causes of excessive absorption
  - Hypervitaminosis D
  - Milk alkali syndrome

Affected Organs

- Kidney—Nephrocalcinosis (calcium is deposited in tubular epithelium and lumen)
- Lungs—Calcium is deposited in the alveoli
- Stomach—Acid secreting fundal glands show calcium deposition
- Blood vessels—In internal elastic lamina calcium deposition is seen

3

Acute Inflammation

Definition

- It is the local response of living mammalian tissue to injury due to any agent.
- It is a body defense reaction to eliminate/limit the spread of injurious agents.

Injurious Agents

- Physical
- Chemical
- Infective
- Immunological

Signs of Inflammation (Fig. 3.1)

Celsus proposed 4 cardinal signs of inflammation
- Rubor (redness)
- Tumor (swelling)

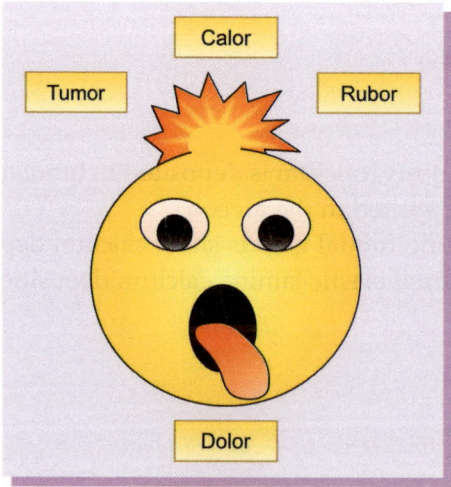

Fig. 3.1: Cardinal signs of inflammation

- Calor (heat)
- Dolor (pain)

Virchow added fifth cardinal sign

- *Functio laesa* (loss of function)

Types of Inflammation

1. Acute Inflammation

It is an early body reaction of short duration and rapid onset.

2. Chronic Inflammation

It may follow after acute inflammation, if acute inflammation persist for long duration or it may be chronic since beginning, and persist for long duration due to stimulus of chronic inflammation.

Acute Inflammation

The process involve two consequent events namely
1. Vascular events
2. Cellular events

1. Vascular Events

The blood vessels show two types of changes
a. Haemodynamic changes
b. Permeability changes

a. Haemodynamic Changes

- Immediately after injury transient vasoconstrictions of arterioles occurs lasting for 3 seconds to 5 minutes. It is followed by
- Persistent progressive vasodilatation that leads to redness (rubor) and increased blood volume in microvascular bed generate warmed (calor).
- Increased local hydrostatic pressure cause transudation of fluid in the interstitium leading to swelling (tumor).
- Slowing of blood flow and stasis leads to movement of leukocyte toward peripheral stream of blood flow known as leukocytic margination.

Haemodynamic changes can be demonstrated by Lewis popular experiment known as "Triple response" characterized by red line, flare and wheal.

b. Permeability Changes

Transudative inflammatory edema due to haemodynamic changes is followed by exudative inflammatory. Edema exudative edema is evident in acute inflammation because of

- Increased vascular permeability so that endothelial lining become leaky
- Osmotic pressure changes

A. Increased vascular permeability changes
   1. Immediate transient vascular permeability response is due to contraction of endothelial cells of venules by histamine and bradykinin.
   2. Prolonged vascular permeability response is due to retraction of endothelial cells due to reorganization of cytoskeleton by IL-1, TNF, in venules.
   3. Delayed prolonged vascular permeability response is due to direct injury to endothelial cells resulting in physical gap in venules, capillaries and arterioles.
   4. Late vascular permeability response is due to injury to endothelium by leukocytes and due to newly formed capillaries (neovascularization) which are leaky.

B. Osmotic pressure changes
   - Intravascular osmotic pressure is decreased.
   - Interstitial osmotic pressure is increased.

Osmotic pressure changes and permeability changes lead to excessive outward flow of fluid from capillaries resulting in exudative inflammatory fluid.

2. Cellular Events

Cellular event consists of:
1. Extravasation of leukocyte
2. Phagocytosis

1. Extravasation of Leukocyte (Fig. 3.2)

It is escape of leukocytes from the lumen of microvasculature to the interstitium. Neutrophils form the 1st line of defense cells followed by monocytes and macrophages.

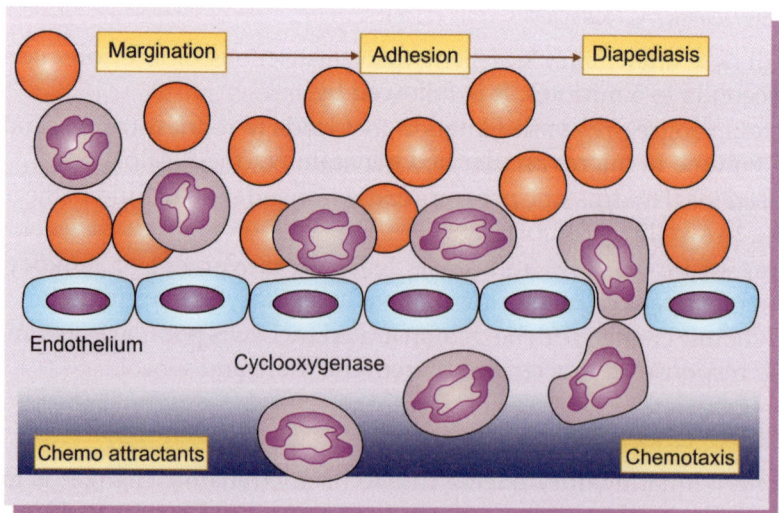

Fig. 3.2: Leukocytic events in acute inflammation

A. Sequence of events in blood vessels (margination)
- Stasis of blood in vessel leads to
- Loss of axial flow of blood cells, resulting in
- Margination of leukocytes and
- Pavement of leukocytes over endothelium

B. Sequence of events over endothelium (adhesion)
- Neutrophils stick briefly to endothelium and roll over it
- Injury to endothelium leads to neutralization of negative charges so that loose adhesion of leukocytes and endothelium is formed
- Later on tight adhesion is brought about by adhesion molecules like
  a. Selectin (P-selectin, E-selectin, L-selectin)
  b. Addressin (leukocytic and endothelial)
  c. Integrin (B1 and B2 molecules)
  d. Immunoglobulin and super family adhesion molecules (ICAM1, 2) intercellular adhesion molecule

C. Sequence of events across endothelium (diapediasis)
- After adhesion leukocytes move along endothelium, they send cytoplasmic pseudopods followed by secretion of collagenase enzyme
- Collagenase dissolves the basement membrane and leukocytes reach in extravascular space
- Basement membrane is repaired immediately
- Within 1st 24 hours neutrophils (short lived) and later on with in 24–48 hours Monocytes and macrophages reach in extravascular space

D. Sequence of events in extravascular space (chemotaxis)
- The chemical which guide the movement of leukocytes are known as chemotactic factors or chemokines
- Transmigration of leukocytes mediated by chemotactic factors across endothelium, basement membrane, perivascular myofibroblasts and matrix to reach the interstitium is known as chemotaxis

Chemokines are
- Leukotriene B_4 (LT B_4)
- Platelet factor 4 (PF4)
- Complement (C5a)
- Cytokines (IL-8)
- Soluble bacterial products
- Monocytic chemoattractant protein
- Chemotactic factor for CD-4 + T cells
- Eotaxin for eosinophils

Specific receptors are present over leukocytes which receive signal from chemokines and leukocytes get activated.

Activated leukocytes
- Produce arachidonic acid metabolites
- Discharge its granules (degranulation)
- Secrete lysosomal enzyme
- Generate oxygen metabolites
- Increase intracellular Ca^{++}
- Increase leukocyte adhesion molecules

2. Phagocytosis

It is the process of engulfment of solid particulate material by phagocytic cells. (Polymorphonuclear cells and macrophages)

Steps of phagocytosis

a. **Opsonization**

Coating of microorganisms by opsonin takes place.

Opsonins are naturally occurring factors present in serum as follows:
- Immunoglobulin: Fc fragment of immunoglobulin is recognized by receptors present on polymorphonuclear cells and macrophages
- Complement: C3b receptors are present on phagocytes

b. **Engulfment**
- Pseudopods are formed around particle, followed by phagocytic vacuole (phagosome) formation by fusion of intervening membrane of pseudopods
- Fusion of lysosomes and phagosome leads to phagolysosome formation

c. **Secretion**
- Preformed granule and stored products of polymorphonuclear cells are discharged in phagolysosome
- In neutrophils azurophilic granules and specific granules are discharged in phagolysosome
- In monocytes arachidonic acid metabolites and oxygen metabolites are released

d. **Degradation**

Killing or digestion of microorganisms takes place by degradation of hydrolytic enzymes. Various mechanism involved are:

I. *Oxygen dependent bactericidal mechanism*
Following oxygen metabolites kills the bacteria

O_2^-, H_2O_2, OH^-, HOCl, HOI, HOBr

$$2O_2 \xrightarrow{\hspace{3cm}} 2O_2^-$$
$$\text{NADPH} \qquad \text{NADP} + H^+$$

$$2O_2^- + 2H^+ \longrightarrow 2H_2O_2$$

a. Myeloperoxidase (MPO) dependent killing by neutrophils and monocytes

$$H_2O_2 \xrightarrow[\text{Cl}^-\ \text{Br}^-\text{I}^-]{\text{MPO}} HOCl + H_2O$$

HOCl is a potent antibacterial agent

b. Myeloperoxidase (MPO) independent killing by mature macrophages

$$H_2O_2 \xrightarrow[\text{Haber-Weiss reaction}]{O_2^-} OH^-$$

$$H_2O_2 \xrightarrow[\text{Fantom reaction}]{Fe^{++}} OH^-$$

II. *Oxygen independent killing mechanism*

Following agents released do not require oxygen

- Hydrolase
- Permeability increasing factors
- Cationic proteins

III. *Nitric oxide mechanism*

- Nitric oxide (NO) produced by endothelial cells and activated macrophages has anti-parasitic and fungicidal action

INFLAMMATORY CELLS

1. Circulating leukocytes
2. Plasma cells
3. Tissue macrophages

1. Circulating Leukocytes

Leukocytes which are present in blood circulation

a. Polymorphonuclear Cells (Neutrophils)

In acute inflammation neutrophils are increased in blood and tissue. Neutrophil granules contain

- Proteases
- MPO
- Lysozyme
- Esterase
- Aryl sulphatase

- Alkaline phosphatase
- Cationic proteins

Functions

- Neutrophils are responsible for initial phagocytosis
- Engulfment of antigen-antibody complex
- Harmful effects are destruction of basement membrane

b. Eosinophils

Granules of eosinophils contain
- Cationic proteins
- Basic proteins
- Enzymes same as neutrophils except lysozyme

Eosinophils are increased in blood and tissues in:
- Allergic conditions
- Parasitic infestations
- Skin diseases
- Lymphoma

c. Basophil-Similar to Mast Cells

Granules of basophil contain
- Heparin
- Histamine

Function

Immediate and delayed hypersensitivity reactions are mediated through heparin and histamine.

d. Lymphocytes

- Blood
- Spleen, thymus, lymph nodes
- MALT (mucosa associated lymphoid tissue)

Function–Lymphocytes

- Activate chronic inflammation
- Stimulate antibody formation
- Confer cell mediated immunity

2. Plasma Cells

Plasma cell is not found in circulating blood or in plasma (contrary to the name).

Plasma cells synthesize immunoglobulin (antibody). Plasma cells are increased in
- Prolonged infection with immunological response
- Hypersensitivity states
- Multiple myeloma

3. Tissue Macrophages (Mononuclear phagocytic/Reticuloendothelial system)

Tissue macrophages are found in tissue and designated by different names at different sites, such as
- Monocytes in the blood
- Macrophages in the tissue
- Histiocytes in connective tissue
- Kupffer cells in liver
- Alveolar macrophages in lungs
- Present in sinusoidal lining of spleen, lymph node, bone marrow
- Present as serous cavity lining
- Microgleal cells in nervous system
- Langerhans' cells of skin
- Dendritic cells in lymph node

Functions of mononuclear phagocytic cells are:
A. Phagocytosis (engulfment of particulate material)
B. Pinocytosis (engulfment of liquid material)
C. Liberate biologically active substances like
  - Protease (collagenase, elastase)
  - Plasminogen activator
  - Products of complements
  - Coagulation factors
  - Chemotactic agents
  - Arachidonic acid metabolites
  - Growth promoting factors for fibroblasts, blood vessels and granulocytes
  - Cytokines
  - Oxygen derived free radicals

4. Giant Cells

When macrophages fail to phagocytose injurious agent, they fuse to form multinucleated giant cells. Various types of giant cells are:

a. Foreign body giant cells. Up to 100 nuclei are seen scattered throughout the cytoplasm, for example, foreign body granuloma

b. Langhans' type giant cells. These are formed in chronic infective granuloma like leprosy and tuberculosis. Numerous nuclei are seen in cytoplasm, arranged in horse-shoe shape manner.

c. Tuton giant cells. Multiple nuclei are seen in vacuolated cytoplasm. For example in xanthoma.
d. Tumor giant cells. Nuclei are atypical and hyperchromatic formed from dividing neoplastic cell. For examples, carcinoma of liver, soft tissue tumors
e. Miscellaneous. Multiple nuclei are seen in mesodermal cells. For example, Aschoff cells in rheumatic nodule, Reed-Sternberg cells in Hodgkin's lymphoma, osteoclasts in osteoclastoma.

CHEMICAL MEDIATORS OF INFLAMMATION (ENDOGENOUS MEDIATORS)

Chemical substances which mediate the tissue response to injury, i.e. inflammation are known as chemical mediators. Various functions performed by chemical mediators are:
• Increase permeability
• Vasodilatation
• Chemotaxis
• Fever, pain, tissue damage

Classifications

A. Cell derived mediators, i.e. mediators released by cells
B. Plasma derived mediators, i.e. mediators originating from plasma

A. Cell Derived Mediators (Fig. 3.3)

   1. Vasoactive amines (histamine, serotonin)

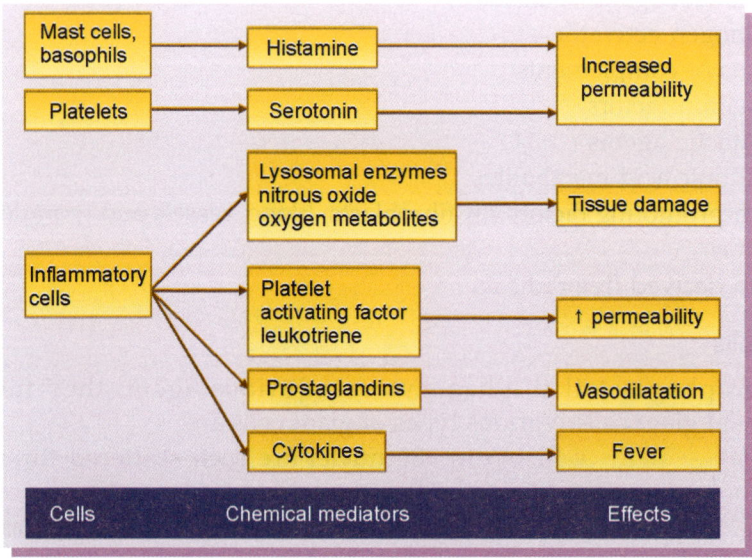

Fig. 3.3: Cell derived chemical mediators

2. Arachidonic acid metabolites (prostaglandin, leukotriene)
3. Lysosomal enzymes
4. Platelet activating factors
5. Cytokines
6. Nitrous oxide
7. Oxygen derived free radicals

1. Vasoactive Amines

A. *Histamine*

It is responsible for early inflammatory response.

Sources

Stored in granules of mast cells, basophils and platelets. Stimulating agents which leads to degranulation and release of histamine are:
- Stimuli causing acute inflammation
- Anaphylotoxins (C3a, C5a)
- Histamine releasing factors from neutrophils, monocytes, platelets
- Neuropeptides substance P)

Action
- Vasodilatation
- Increase vascular permeability
- Itching, pain

B. *5-Hydroxytryptamine (5-HT or Serotonin)*

Sources

Stored in chromaffin cells of GIT, spleen, nervous tissue, mast cells and platelets

Action

Similar to histamine but it is less potent than histamine

2. Arachidonic Acid Metabolites (Fig. 3.4)

Sources

These are substances synthesized during metabolic degradation of arachidonic acid and are classified into two types.

 I. Leukotriens
II. Prostaglandins
- All leukocytes produce leukotriene
- All leukocytes, platelets and endothelial cells produce prostaglandins

Synthesis
- Lipoxygenase pathway
  - Arachidonic acid produces various leukotrienes like LTC_4, LTB_4, LTD_4, and LTF_4 through lipoxygenase pathway

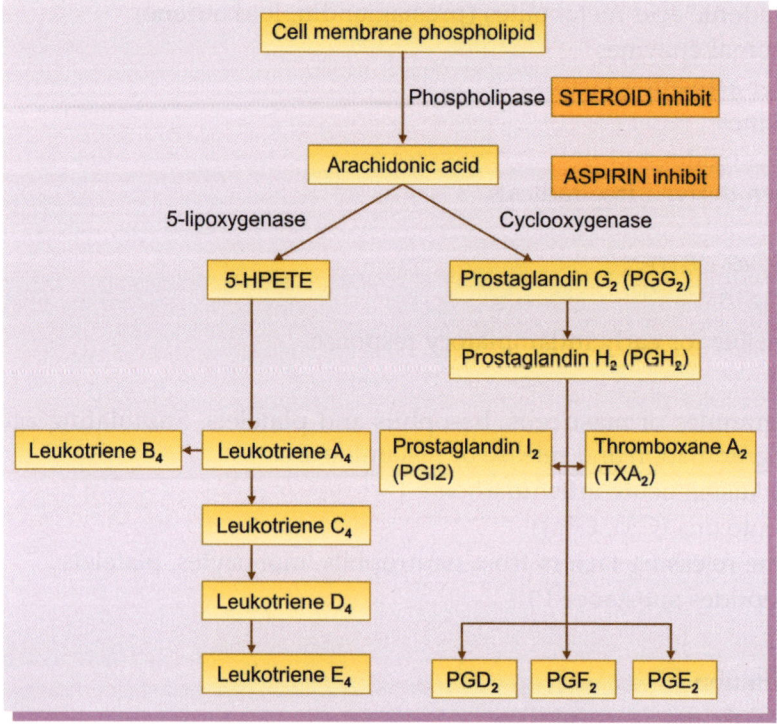

Fig. 3.4: Arachidonic acid metabolites

- Cyclooxygenase pathway
  – Prostaglandin like substances like PGD_2, PGE_2, PGF_2, PGI_2 and thromboxane (TXA_2) are produced through cyclooxygenase pathway.

Actions of Leukotrienes
- LTB_4
  – Chemotactic for phagocytic cells
  – Stimulate phagocytic cells adherence
- LTC_4, LTD_4, LTE_4
  – Smooth muscle contraction leading to vasoconstriction and bronchoconstriction.
  – Increase vascular permeability

Actions of Prostaglandins
- PGD_2 and PGE_2
  – Vasodilatation and bronchodilatation
  – Increases permeability
- PGF_2
  – Vasodilatation and bronchoconstriction

- Thromboxan (TXA$_2$)
  - Platelet aggregation
  - Bronchoconstriction and vasoconstriction
- PGI$_2$
  - Vasodilatation and bronchodilatation
  - Anti-platelet aggregating agent
- Aspirin and other anti-inflammatory drugs inhibit cyclooxygenase enzyme thereby reducing concentration of prostaglandins
- Steroids inhibit phospholipases enzyme, hence reducing concentration of both leukotriens and prostaglandins

3. *Lysosomal Enzymes*

Sources

Neutrophils and monocytes contain lysosomal granules

In neutrophils

Specific (secondary) lysosomal granules contain following enzymes:
- Lactoferrin
- Lysozyme
- Alkaline phosphatase
- Collagenase

Azurophilic (primary) lysosomal granules contain following enzymes:
- Myeloperoxidase
- Acid hydrolase
- Neutral proteases (elastase)
- Collagenase
- Proteinase

In monocytes lysosomal granules contain following enzymes:
- Acid proteases
- Collagenase
- Elastase
- Plasminogen activators

4. *Platelet Activating Factors*

Sources

Platelet activating factors are released from IgE activated basophils/mast cells leukocytes, endothelium, and platelets

Action

Platelet activating factor cause
- Platelet aggregation

- Increase vascular permeability
- Vasodilatation in low and vasoconstriction in high concentration
- Bronchoconstriction
- Adherence of leukocytes to endothelium
- Chemotaxis

5. Cytokines

Cytokines are proteins produced by many cell types that modulate the function of other cell type. These are of two types:
1. Interleukins and TNF
2. Chemokines

Sources
- Activated lymphocytes produce lymphokins
- Macrophages produce monokins
- Haematopoietic cells produce interleukins

Properties
- Many growth factors act as cytokines while many cytokines act as growth factors
- Cytokines are produced during immune and inflammatory response
- Their receptor regulated effects are transient, pleiotropic and multifunctional

Classification (depending upon function of cytokines)
- Cytokines which regulates lymphocytic functions are:
  - IL-2, IL-4, which has positive effect on lymphocytes
  - IL-10, TGF-B shows negative effect on lymphocytes
- Cytokines which are involved with natural immunity are:
  - TNF-α, IL-1β, 1FN-α and β, IL-6
- Cytokines which activate inflammatory cells are:
  - INF-γ, TNF-α, TNF-β, IL-5, IL-10, IL-12
- Cytokines which act as chemoattractant for neutrophil are chemokines
- Cytokines which stimulate haematopoiesis are:
  - IL-3, IL-7, C-Kit legend, GM-CSF, M-CSF, stem cell factor

1. Interleukins and TNF
Endotoxins, immune complex, toxins and physical injury stimulate macrophages and lymphocytes to produce interleukins and TNF. Activated macrophages produce IL-1, TNF-α, activated T cell produce TNF-α and IL-γ. The effects may be:
- Autocrine, i.e. stimulating to self
- Paracrine, i.e. stimulating other cells in the vicinity
- Endocrine, i.e. stimulating distant cells carried via blood

Actions of interleukin and TNF

A. Local acute phase reaction. It involves

1. Endothelium activation resulting in
   - Adhesion molecule synthesis
   - Chemical mediator synthesis
   - Matrix modulating enzyme synthesis
   - Increased thrombogenicity
2. Leukocytic aggregation and priming
3. Fibroblastic proliferation and collagen synthesis

B. Systemic acute phase response leads to

Fever, decrease appetite, decrease blood pressure, increased heart rate, release of ACTH and corticosteroid, decrease vascular resistance, decrease pH, slow wave sleep, and leukocytosis

C. Control of body mass

It has been seen that if TNF-α, action is impaired obesity develops and TNF-α, over production cause cachexia.

2. *Chemokines*

Properties

These are 8–10 KD proteins which act as activator and chemoattractant for leukocytes. It is composed of small protein with paired cysteine repeat and two internal disulfide bridges.

Classification of chemokines is based on arrangement of cysteine residue

1. C-X-C (α-chemokines): Two cysteine residues are separated by cysteine residue. For example, IL-8. IL-8 is secreted by activated macrophages and endothelium. It acts on neutrophils.
2. C-C (β-chemokines): Two cysteine residues are adjacent to each other. For example, MIP-1α, MIP-1β, MCP-1, 2, 3. These chemokines are chemotactic for monocytes. Eotaxin is chemotactic for eosinophils.
3. C (γ-chemokines): It lacks first and third cysteine residue, e.g. lymphotactin which attracts lymphocytes.
4. CX_3C (fractalkines): Three amino acids are present between two cysteine residues. Its surface bound form induces adhesion of monocytes and T cells and its soluble form is chemoattractant for monocytes.

Action

Chemokines act on stromal cells and get bound with them. It results in immobilization of chemokines. Thus chemokines maintain chemotactic gradient for chemotaxis.

6. Nitrous Oxide

Source
Nitrous oxide is produced by macrophages, endothelial cells and neuronal cells

Action
- Nitrous oxide causes vasodilatation by relaxing vascular musculature and has paracrine effect because of short half-life
- It has antimicrobial action also

Synthesis
Nitrous oxide is synthesized by the action of nitrous oxide synthetase enzyme.
- Endothelial cells contain e NOS (nitrous oxide synthetase)
- Macrophages contain i NOS (nitrous oxide synthetase)
- Neurons contain n NOS (nitrous oxide synthetase)

They can produce nitrous oxide by acting with L-arginine, oxygen, NADP and co factors. Activity of e NOS and n NOS is dependent on free calcium and cytokines.

Mechanism of action
Nitrous oxide induce cyclic GMP which causes relaxation of smooth muscle cell (short duration) and form a complex with thiol group of proteins (stable form).

Effects of nitrous oxide are
1. Vasodilatation
2. Decrease platelet aggregation, adhesion and degranulation
3. Decrease leukocyte recruitment
4. Decrease mast cell induced inflammation

7. Oxygen Derived Free Radicals

Source
O_2 derived free radicals are O_2^-, H_2O_2, OH^- produced by neutrophil and macrophages

Actions
1. Low level release cause
   - Increase expressions of chemokines
   - Endothelial–leukocytic adhesions
2. High level release cause
   - Endothelial cell damage leading to increased permeability
   - Inactivation of anti proteases
   - Injury to other cells

Antioxidants which protect against free radical induced damage are:
- Ceruloplasmin
- Transferrin
- Superoxide dismutase (SOD)

- Catalase
- Glutathione peroxidase

B. *Plasma Derived Mediators* (Fig. 3.5)

Various products derived from activation and interaction of 4 interlinked systems in plasma also mediate inflammation. These are:

1. Kinin system
2. Clotting system
3. Fibrinolytic system
4. Complement system
   - Hageman factor (factor XII) plays a key role in interaction of these four systems
   - Glass, basement membrane, kaolin, bacterial endotoxins activate factor XII
   - Factor XII in turn activates fibrinolytic system, clotting system and kinin system which produce plasmin, fibrin/fibrin split product and bradykinin
   - These activate ultimately complement, so that C3a and C5a (permeability factors) are released

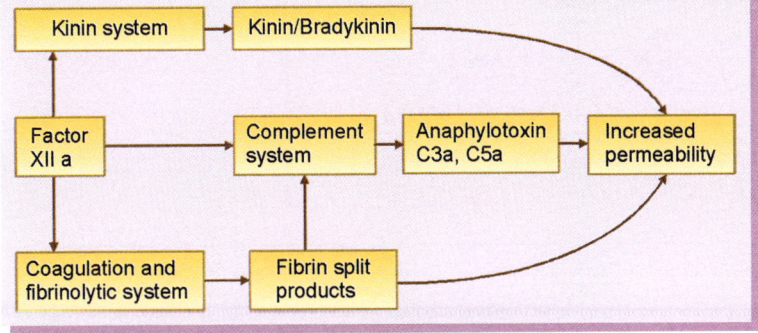

Fig. 3.5: Plasma derived chemical mediators

1. *Kinin System* (Fig. 3.6)

Actions of bradykinin are:
- Smooth muscle contraction
- Vasodilatation, increased permeability
- Pain

2. *Clotting System* (Fig. 3.7)

3. *Fibrinolytic System*

Actions of thrombin and fibrin split products
- Leukocytic adhesion enhancement

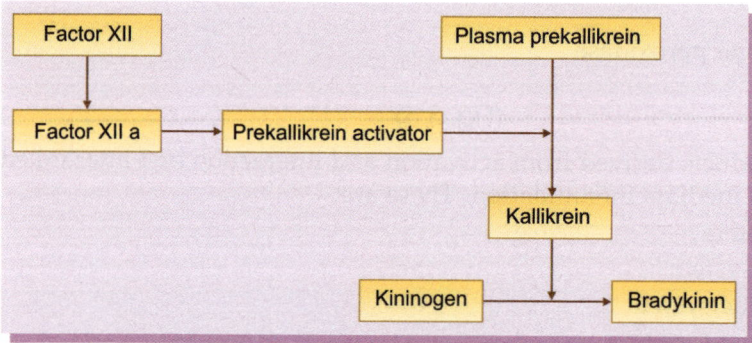

Fig. 3.6: Kinin system

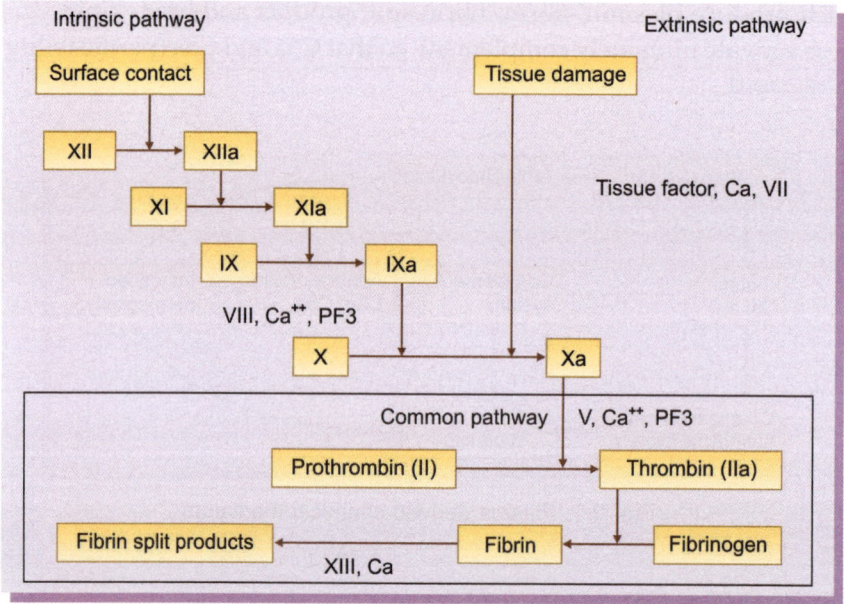

Fig. 3.7: Coagulation and fibrinolytic system

- Increased capillary permeability
- Chemotaxis of neutrophils

4. Complement System (Fig. 3.8)

Actions of C3a, C4a, C5a
- Release histamine
- Increase permeability
- C3b augment phagocytosis

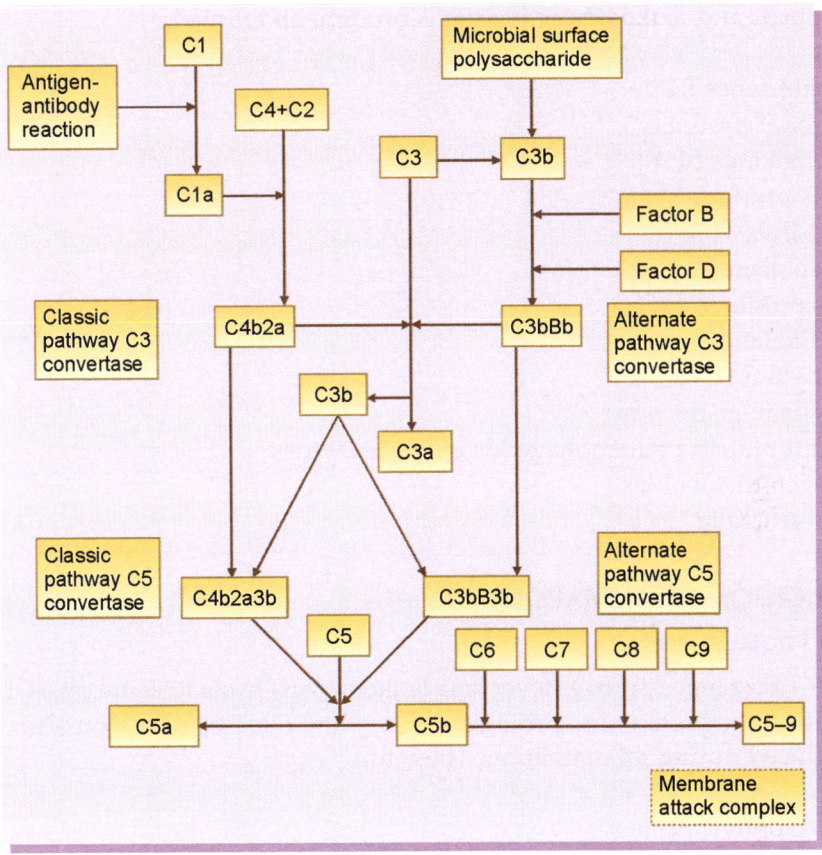

Fig. 3.8: Compliment activation pathway

- C5a is chemotactic for leukocytes
- Membrane attack complex (MAC) makes a pore in cell membrane of invading microorganism

CHEMICAL MEDIATORS AND THEIR EFFECT (Fig. 3.3)

1. Vasodilatation is produced by
   - Prostaglandin and
   - Nitrous oxide
2. Vascular permeability is increased by
   - Vasoactive amines
   - C3a, C5a
   - Bradykinin
   - Leukotrienes C4 D4 E4
   - Platelet activating factors

3. Chemotaxis and leukocyte activation is brought about by
   - C5a
   - Leukotrienes B4
   - Bacterial products
   - Chemokines (IL-8)
4. Fever is produced by
   - IL-1, IL-6, TNF
   - Prostaglandin
5. Pain is produced by
   - Prostaglandin
   - Bradykinin
6. Tissue damage done by
   - Neutrophil and macrophage lysosomal enzymes
   - Oxygen metabolites
   - Nitrous oxide

REGULATION OF INFLAMMATION

1. **Acute Phase Proteins**
   - APP + Systemic features (fever and leukocytosis) leads to acute phase response.
   - Acute phase proteins are produced in liver and released in response to cytokines produced during inflammation. These are
   - α-1 antitrypsin
   - α-1 acid glycoprotein
   - Protease inhibitor
   - Hepatoglobin
   - Reactive protein
   - Serum amyloid-A
   - P Component

   Deficiency of APP leads to severe disease, chronicity and recurrences.

2. **Corticosteroids** provide self regulated anti-inflammatory response.

3. **Free Cytokine Receptors** regulate inflammation.

4. **Suppressor T cells** inhibit function of T and B cells.

5. **Anti-inflammatory mediators** like PGE_2 and PGI_2 regulate by opposing action.

MORPHOLOGICAL TYPES OF ACUTE INFLAMMATION

Inflammation of an organ is named by adding suffix "tis" to the Latin name. For example:
- Inflammation of appendix   Appendicitis
- Inflammation of testis   Orchitis
- Inflammation of liver   Hepatitis

- Inflammation if tonsils   Tonsillitis
- Inflammation of tongue   Glossitis

Types

1. Serous Inflammation

It is characterized by collection of watery low protein content fluid derived from plasma or serous lining of serous cavities. For example, burn, viral vesicle

2. Fibrinous Inflammation (Fig. 3.9)

Deposition of fibrin at inflammatory site is known as fibrinous inflammation. It is seen in case of severe injury.

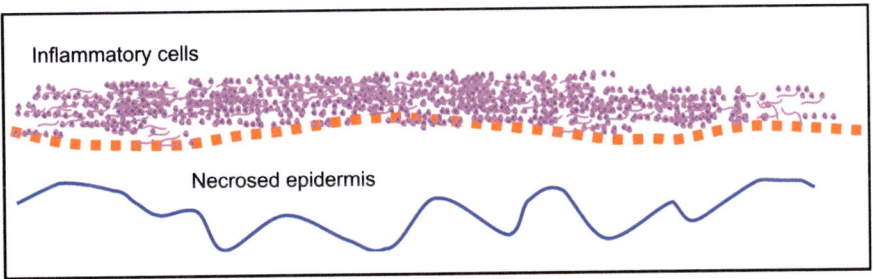

Fig. 3.9: Fibrinous inflammation

3. Pseudomembranous Inflammation

Inflammation of mucus membrane with diphtheria leads to necrosis of mucosa by diphtheria toxins. Denuded epithelium and plasma form a membrane (false membrane) hence the name.

4. Suppuration (Abscess formation) (Fig. 3.10)

Intense inflammation leads to collection of neutrophils, necrotic debris and edematous fluid forming purulent exudative fluid. It is seen in inflammation associated with pyogenic bacteria. For example, boils, carbuncle, furuncle. When collected in a closed cavity, it results in abscess formation.

5. Ulcer (Fig. 3.11)

Breech in the continuity of skin or mucus membrane is called ulcer. For example, typhoid, tuberculosis, amoebiasis, varicose ulcer.

6. Cellulitis

It is spreading soft tissue inflammation, because of hyaluronidase enzyme released by some bacteria. Hyaluronidase facilitates the spread on inflammation faster.

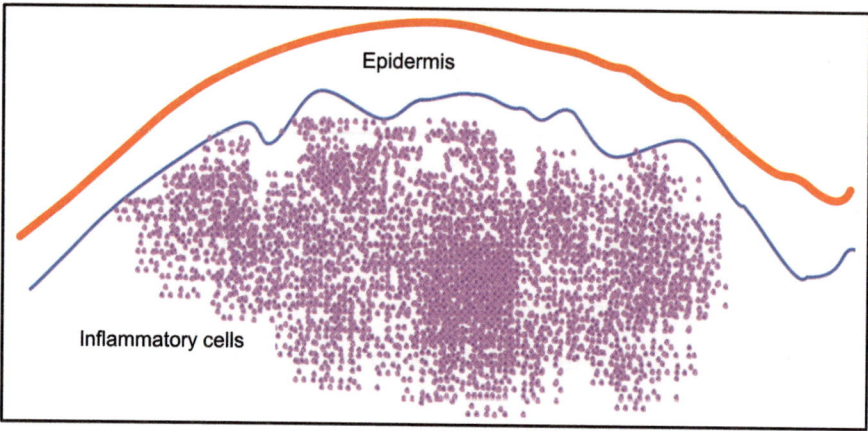

Fig. 3.10: Suppurative inflammation

7. Bacterial Infections of Blood

Blood is a liquid tissue, therefore inflammation leads systemic effects. Injurious agents may reach to the circulation directly from environment of from any other lesion at different site.

i. Bacteraemia

Small numbers of bacteria are present in blood. They do not multiply significantly and are not detected by microscopy. For example, *S. typhi, E. coli, S. viridans*

ii. Septicemia

Rapidly multiplying highly pathogenic bacteria are present in blood. For example, pyogenic streptococci. It is accompanied by systemic effect like toxemia, multiple small hemorrhages, neutrophilic leukocytosis, DIC.

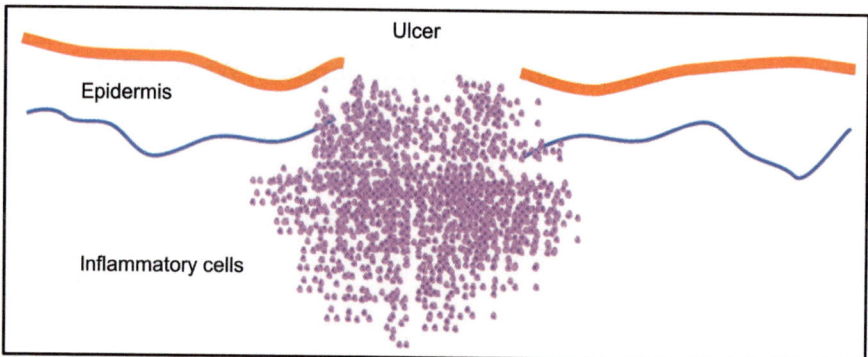

Fig. 3.11: Ulcerative inflammation

iii. *Pyaemia*

Dissemination of small septic thrombi is present in blood which cause their effect where they are lodged. For example,

a. Pyaemic abscess—necrosis in centre surrounded by bacteria, suppurations and acute inflammatory cell.
b. Septic infarcts—large thrombi leads to infarction of lung, liver, brain and kidney.

SYSTEMIC EFFECT OF INFLAMMATION

Local tissue responses are accompanied by systemic effect.

1. Fever

- Due to bacteraemia
- Because of prostaglandin, IL-1 and TNF

2. Leukocytosis

Increased leukocyte count is seen in different infections, e.g.
- Bacterial infection Neutrophilia
- Viral infection Lymphocytosis
- Parasitic infection Eosinophilia

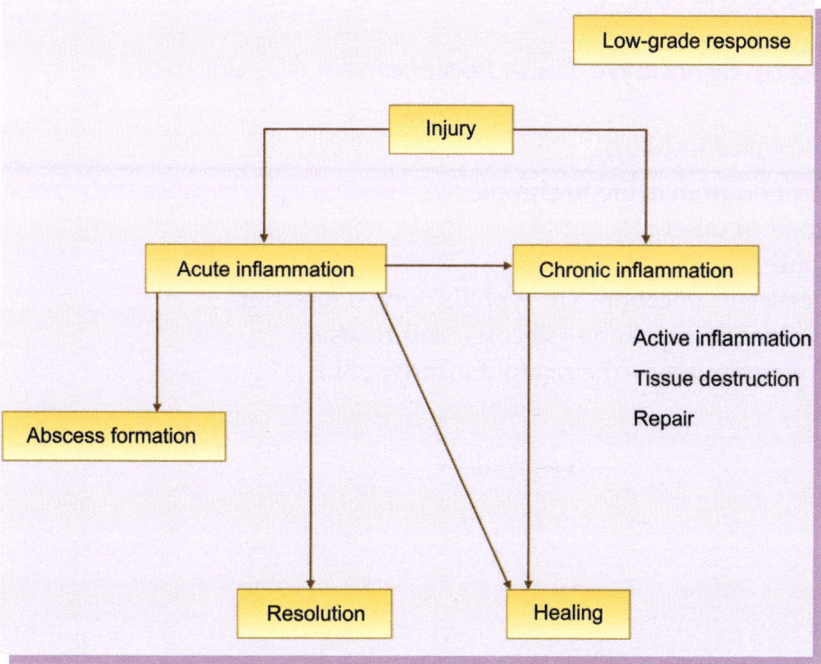

Fig. 3.12: Outcome of acute inflammation

3. Lymphangiitis and Lymphadenitis

Lymphatics and lymph nodes draining the inflamed tissue shows reactive inflammatory charges, because of chemical mediator released from inflamed tissue. Lymph node shows follicular hyperplasia and sinus histiocytosis.

4. Shock

Massive release of cytokines, TNF-L cause profuse vasodilatation, increase vascular permeability and decrease intravascular volume leading to shock which activate coagulation pathway and results in bleeding and death because of DIC and micro thrombi formation.

OUTCOME OF ACUTE INFLAMMATION

1. Complete Resolution

- Neutralization and spontaneous decay of chemical mediators
- Return of normal permeability
- Decrease neutrophilic infiltrate
- Death of neutrophils (apoptosis)
- Removal of edema fluid, proteins leukocytes, foreign agents, necrotic debris from the site.

2. Abscess Formation (Pyogenic organisms)

3. Healing by Connective Tissue Replacement (Organization)

4. Chronic Inflammation

- Transition from acute to chronic
- Chronic at onset
  Because of
  a. Persistent infection, TB, syphilis, fungal infection
  b. Prolonged exposure—silicosis, anthrocosis
  c. Autoimmunity—rheumatoid arthritis, SLE

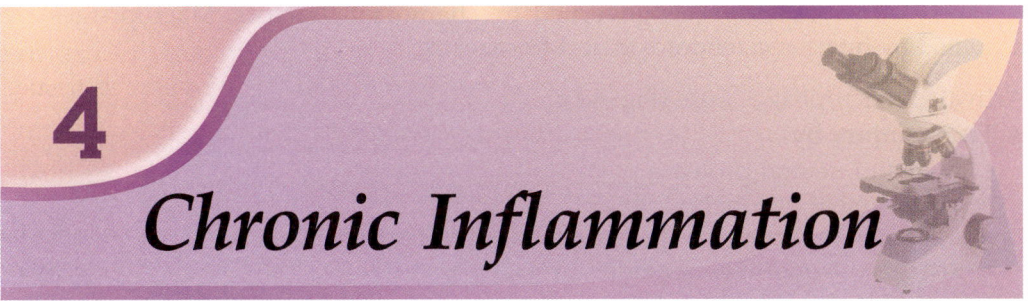

4

Chronic Inflammation

Definition

It is defined as inflammation of prolonged duration, in which active inflammation, tissue injury and healing proceed simultaneously.

Characteristic Features

- Mononuclear infiltrate is composed of lymphocytes, macrophages and plasma cells
- Tissue destruction
- Repair, i.e. angiogenesis and fibrosis

Types

1. Acute inflammation progresses to chronic inflammation, because of
   - Persistence of injurious agent
   - Interference in normal process of healing. For example, peptic ulcer
2. Chronic inflammation, since beginning when
   - Caused by less noxious injurious agent
   - Inflammation fails to resolve. For example,
     a. Viral infections
     b. Microbial infection (TB, syphilis, fungal)
     c. Toxic agents (non-degradable)
        - Exogenous—silica
        - Endogenous—atherosclerosis
     d. Autoimmune diseases
        - Self antigen induces perpetuating immunological reaction

CHRONIC INFLAMMATORY CELLS

1. Macrophages

Macrophages are monocytes in blood stream. Macrophages are labeled by different names in the tissue. For example:

- Kupffer cells in liver
- Sinus histiocytes in lymph node
- Alveolar macrophages in lung

Migration of macrophage is governed by chemotactic factors. Macrophages are activated by interferon, endotoxin and fibronectin.

Activated macrophage cause (Fig. 4.1):

A. **Tissue injury by**
- Acid and neutral protease
- Complement products C_1 to C_5
- Coagulation factors like properdin, V, VIII and tissue factors
- Reactive O_2 and nitrous oxide
- Arachidonic acid metabolites

B. **Fibrosis by**
- Growth factor
- Fibrogenic cytokines
- Angiogenesis inducing agents
- Remodeling collagenase

2. Lymphocytes

Mobilization of lymphocytes takes place by
- Immune stimuli like antibody mediated and cell mediated
- Nonimmune stimuli like trauma and infarction

Macrophage–Lymphocyte Interaction (Fig. 4.2)

Lymphocytes when activated, convert macrophages, into the activated macrophages with the help of γ-interferon. Activated macrophage secretes cytokines (IL-1) which regulate T lymphocyte activity.

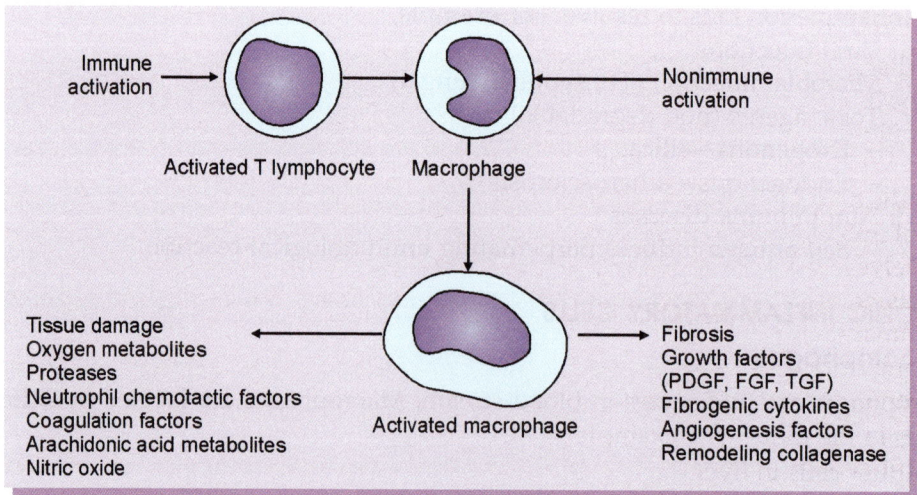

Fig. 4.1: Action of macrophage other than phagocytosis

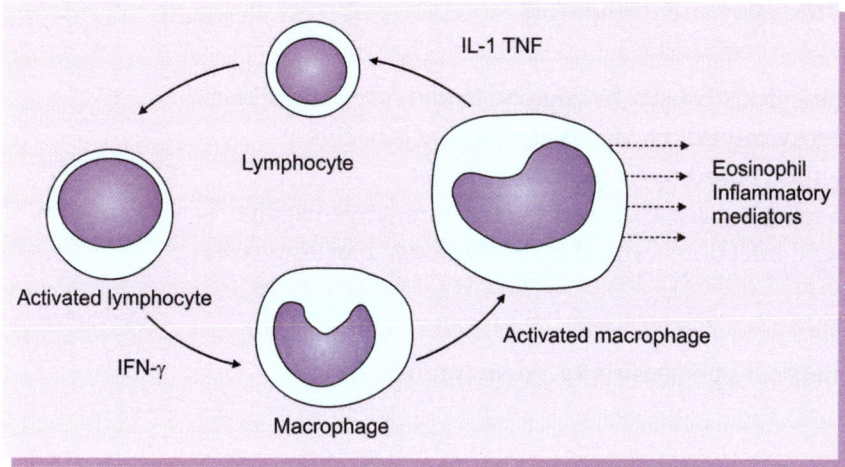

Fig. 4.2: Lymphocyte-macrophage interaction

3. Eosinophils

Eosinophils move in response to chemotactic factor eotaxin (cytokine) released from leukocytes and epithelial cells. These cells are involved in IgE mediated immune reaction and parasitic infections. Eosinophils contain major basic protein which is highly toxic to parasite and epithelial cells.

4. Mast Cells

Mast cells express receptors for Fc portion of IgE antibody and release mediators when it binds with Fc portion of IgE.

GRANULOMATOUS INFLAMMATIONS

It is a distinct chronic granulomatous inflammation characterized by focal accumulation of modified macrophages, because of persistent T cell response. For example, tuberculosis, syphilis, fungus and foreign body.

It is Wall off Phenomenon, to check further spread of infection, if body is not able to eradicate or kill the causal organism. Granulomatous inflammation is a specific kind of inflammation seen in certain chronic infections, in which macrophages modify themselves into epithelioid cell (epithelial cell like), to prevent spread of causative organisms by forming a granule like structure, hence, known as granulomatous inflammation.

Along with granule formation lymphocytic infiltrate and peculiar type of giant cells are seen in the vicinity, which is further surrounded by fibroblastic tissue (reparative process) (Fig. 4.3).

Giant cells are formed as an effort to kill causative organism, by fusion of many epithelioid cells or by continuous nuclear division without cytoplasmic division (Fig. 4.4).

Etiological Types of Granuloma

A. Infectious Granuloma

- Tuberculosis caused by *Mycobacterium tuberculosis* bacilli
- Leprosy caused by *Mycobacterium leprae* bacilli
- Syphilis caused by *Treponema pallidum*
- Cat scratch disease caused by gram-negative bacilli
- Fungal infections caused by *Histoplasma*, blastomycosis

B. Noninfectious Granuloma (Immune Granuloma)

Sarcoidosis, hypersensitivity pneumonitis

C. Foreign Body Granuloma

Due to talc, suture, foreign body, which get buried in the tissue.

Morphological Features

- Aggregated epithelioid cells with pink granular cytoplasm and distinct cell borders
- Surrounded by lymphocytic infiltrate

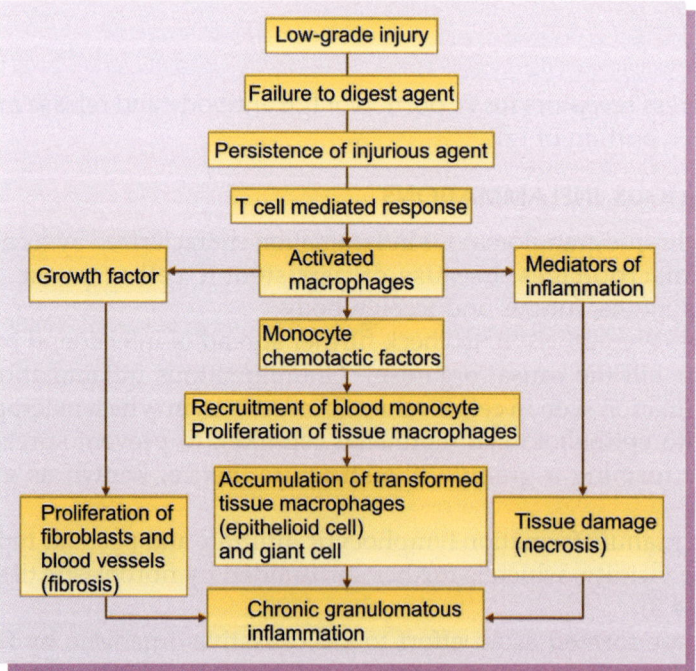

Fig. 4.3: Mechanism of granuloma formation

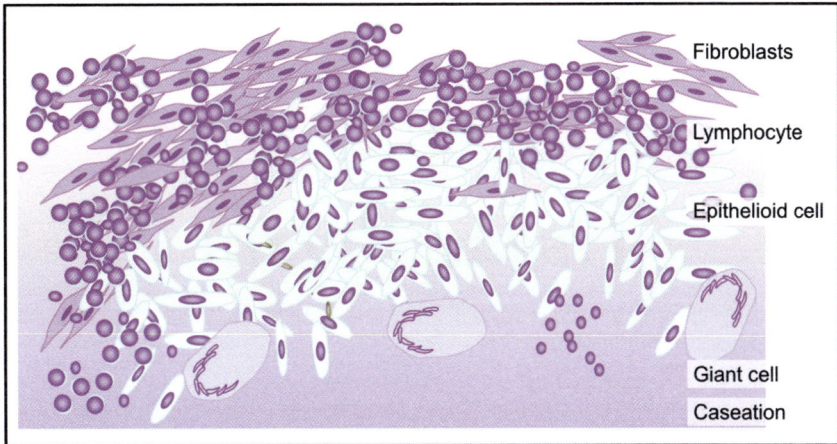

Fig. 4.4: Chronic granulomatous inflammation

- Fibroblasts in older lesions
- Frequent giant cells (fused epithelioid cells forming large cell with more than 20 nuclei in cytoplasm)
- Caseous amorphous necrosis

Morphological Types of Granuloma

1. Serous Granulomatous Inflammation

Protein poor fluid is collected in serous cavities from serum or secretion from mesothelial cells

2. Fibrinous Granulomatous Inflammation

Severe injury causes fibrinogen to pass out and form fibrin meshwork or clot. If lesion do not resolve, it is organized and form scar

3. Suppurative Granulomatous Inflammation

Neutrophils, necrotic cells, and edema fluid get collected to form cold abscess

4. Ulcerative Granulomatous Inflammation

Epithelial structure is necrosed and subepithelium shows acute/chronic inflammation

Systemic Effects

1. Fever
2. Increase somnolence, malaise anorexia
3. Decrease blood pressure
4. Increase ESR
5. Leukocytosis, eosinophilia, lymphocytosis, leucopenia (typhoid, viral)

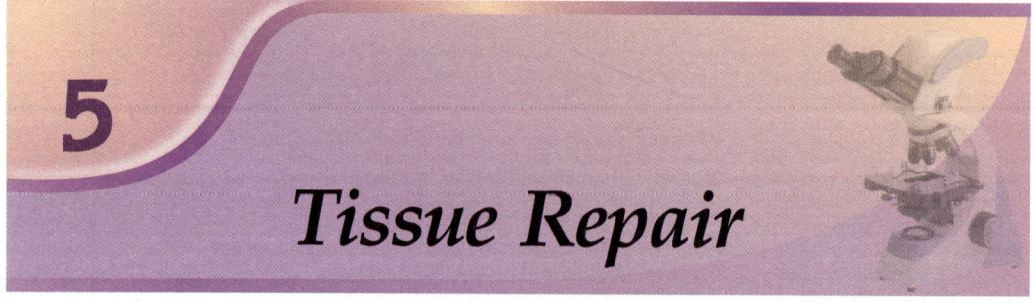

5

Tissue Repair

TISSUE

Tissue is composed of cells and extracellular matrix.

Cell (Fig. 5.1)

Depending on the proliferative potential, the cells may be divided into three types.

1. *Labile Cells*

The cells which remain in continuously dividing state throughout the life are called labile cells. Dead and injured cells are replenished by newer cells continuously. For example, epithelial cells and haematopoietic cells.

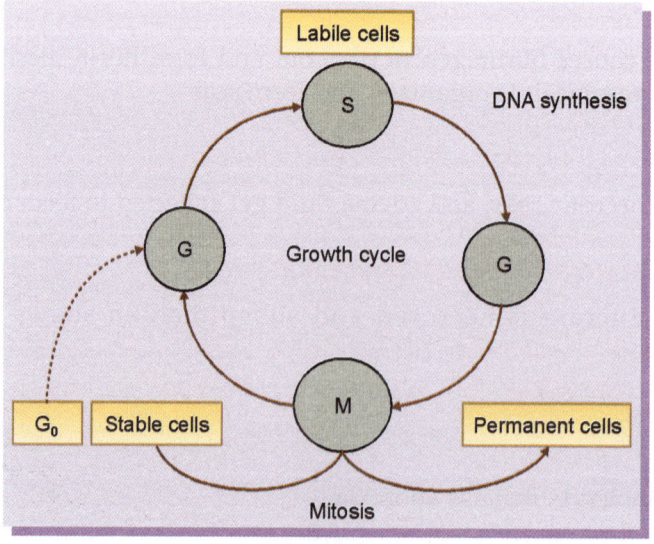

Fig. 5.1: Growth cycle

2. *Stable or Quiescent Cells*

Those cells which do not replicate actively, but they are capable to proliferate in response to tissue damage are known as stable or quiescent cells. Replication of the cells occurs in response to certain stimulants like injury, cell debris, mechanical damage, etc. For example, parenchymal cells of solid organs, endothelial cells, fibroblasts, smooth muscle cells.

3. *Permanent Cells*

Permanent cells are terminally differentiated cells and are not capable of regeneration at all. For example, nerve cells, cardiac cells.

Extracellular Matrix (ECM)

It consists of
1. Fibrous structural protein (collagen, elastin).
2. Gel of proteoglycans and hyaluronan.
3. Adhesive glycoproteins (fibronectin and laminin).

1. *Fibrous Structural Proteins*

Collagen

Collagen is composed of triple helix of 3 polypeptide α-chains, braided into a rope like structure. It is synthesized in ribosomes (Fig. 5.2)

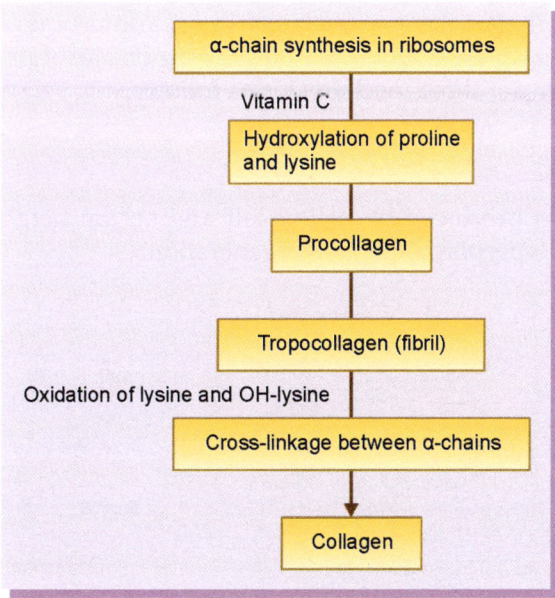

Fig. 5.2: Synthesis of collagen

Elastin, Fibrillin and Elastic Fibre

Blood vessels, skin, uterus required elasticity for their functions. These are made up of elastin. It is synthesized by fibroblast and smooth muscle cells. It has a central core (elastin) and peripheral microfibrillar network (fibrillin).

2. Gel of Proteoglycans and Hyaluronan

It is a made up of a polysaccharide and hyaluronan (monosaccharide). It provides compressibility and serves as reservoir of growth factors.

3. Adhesive Glycoproteins

They provide binding material for cell membrane and extracellular matrix. These are
- *Fibronectin:* It is produced by fibroblasts, monocytes, endothelial cells and connects cells to collagen fibers.
- *Laminin*: It is a glycoprotein in basement membrane of blood vessel. It regulates alignment of endothelial cells and capillary tube formation.
- *Adhesion receptors* (cell adhesion molecules or CAMS). These are immunoglobulin, catherins, selectin and integrin.

CELL GROWTH

Molecular Events

Signal (Fig. 5.3)

The cells grow through signal receptor mechanism. Various types of signals are injury, cell debris, mechanical deformations, etc. Depending on site of production and site of action of signal, there are three mechanisms as follows:

a. Autocrine Signal

Stimulating signal is produced by cells itself and act on neighborhood cells. For example, epithelial hyperplasia, hepatic regeneration.

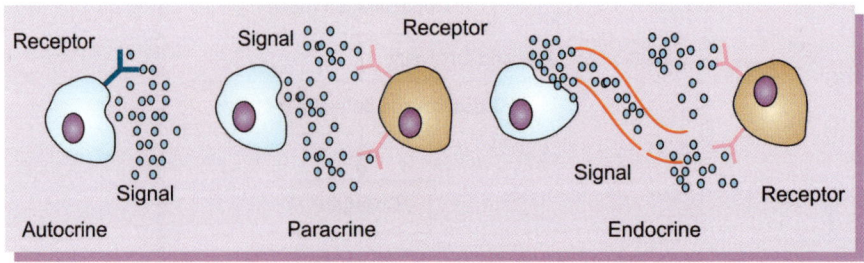

Fig. 5.3: Types of signal

b. *Paracrine Signaling*

Signals are produced by one type of cells and act over other type of cells. For example, in repair macrophage produce signal for fibroblast to proliferate.

c. *Endocrine Signaling*

Stimulating signals are produced by glands which reach to the site of action through circulating blood. For example, TSH released from pituitary gland stimulates thyroid glands.

Receptors

Receptors are surface bound molecules present on target cells, when binds to a legend (signal), it triggers a series of intracellular events to induce transcription factor, activation or repression of activity.

A. *Intrinsic Kinase Receptor*

When stimulated by signal, it activates intracellular proteins like RAS, PI3, PLC-γ. These proteins induce transcription and entry into cell cycle. For example, EGF, TGF-α, PDGF and VEGF.

B. *Nonintrinsic Kinase Receptor*

Stimulated by signal, it activates intranuclear gene transcription through JAK and STAT. For example, IL-2, IL-3, IFN.

C. *G-Protein Linked Receptor*

When stimulated, it activates G-protein resulting in activation of proteins which release calcium from endoplasmic reticulum.

Signal Transduction System

Signal transduction takes place through any one of the following pathways
- MAP (Mitogen activated protein) kinase pathway
- Phosphoinositide – 3 kinase pathway (PI-3)
- Inositol lipid pathway (IP3)

Regulation of Cell Division

Following factors regulate cell division and cell growth,
- Transcription factors: They regulate gene expression in nucleus at transcription level. These factors increase or decrease the expression of gene thereby promoting or inhibiting the cell growth
- Cyclins: These factors regulate protein phosphorylation pathway
- Check points: Check points monitors completion of molecular event

HEALING

Healing is the body response towards injury, an attempt to restore normal structure and function of the tissue.

Regeneration

When healing occurs with the proliferation of same kind of tissue with the restoration of normal histology, it is called regeneration. Labile and stable cells up to certain extent undergo regeneration.

Repair

When healing occurs by proliferation of connective tissue, so that almost normal shape is achieved but specialized function is lacking, it is known as repair. Permanent cells and extensive loss of labile or stable cells heal by repair. Repair involves two events.

Events of Healing

1. Granulation tissue formation: Granulation tissue term is loosely used for the naked eye appearance of tissue, i.e. red granular surface. Microscopically it is composed of proliferating capillaries, fibroblast and thin strands of collagen bundles along with blood and inflammatory cells.
2. Contraction of wound: Contraction of wound occurs after 2 to 3 days after injury. It involves dehydration, contraction of collagen bundles and myofibroblasts.

Healing by First Intension (Primary union)

Clean and uninfected wound with opposed edges (surgical incision) heals by first intension. Surgical incision means limited epithelial cell and connective tissue damage, disruption of basement membrane, space filled with blood and scab formation.

Steps of Healing by 1st Intension (Fig. 5.4)

Immediately	Initial haemorrhage—approximated edges and space between surfaces is filled with blood clot.
In 24 hours	Acute inflammation—neutrophils appear in the margins of wound.
In 48 hours	Epithelization—basal cell layer proliferate and migrate towards incision space known as epithelial spur. Epithelial cell spur migrate to fuse in midline of wound, separating dry scab over surface and necrotic debris with blood clot in dermis. Basement material deposition occur.
By 3rd day	Early organization—neutrophils are replaced by macrophages. Granulation tissue is seen in the incisional space. Vertically oriented collagen fibers are laid down at the margins of incision.
By 5th day	Late organization—neovascularization is at the maximum. Collagen fibers are abundant and bridges incisional gap.

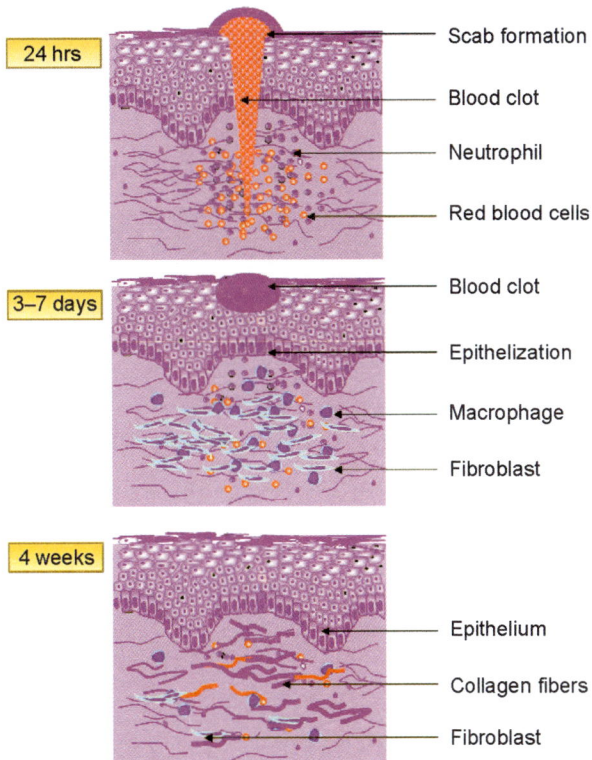

Fig. 5.4: Healing by 1st intension

	Epidermis acquire normal thickness and differentiation of surface cells yield mature epithelial cells
By 1st week	Scar formation—proliferation and accumulation of fibroblasts occur. Leukocytes, edema, increased vascularity, all disappear. In case of surgical wound, sutures are removed on 7th day. Suture track is absorbed.
By 1st month	Scar tissue is covered by intact epidermis get full strength and elasticity. Dermal appendages are destroyed.

Healing by Second Intension (Fig. 5.5)

Healing by secondary intension is seen when there is extensive loss of cells and tissue. For example, infarction, inflammatory ulcerations, abscess. It is characterized by

- Abundant granulation tissue
- More inflammation
- Wound contracture (because of altered fibroblast, i.e. myofibroblasts) which help in bringing cut edges close together
- Substantial scar formation

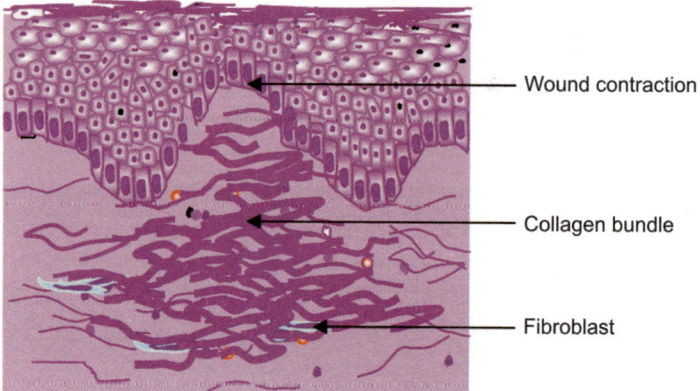

Fig. 5.5: Healing by second intension

Wound Strength

- By the end of 1st week 10% of normal tensile strength is achieved.
- By the end of 3rd month 70–80% of normal tensile strength is achieved

Factors which Delay Wound Healing

Systemic Causes

- Nutrition, vitamin C deficiency
- Altered metabolic state, like diabetes mellitus, malnutrition, obesity
- Altered circulatory state like anaemia, atherosclerosis
- Hormones like glucocorticoids

Local Causes

- Persistence of infection
- Mechanical stress at local site
- Foreign body within the wound
- Large amount of haemorrhage and necrosis

REPAIR BY CONNECTIVE TISSUE

Repair by connective tissue is seen in necrotizing inflammation, accompanied by damage to parenchyma and damage to stromal network. Nondividing cells are destroyed hence repair is made by fibrosis.

Fibrosis is replacement of nonregenerating parenchymal cells by connective tissue.

Steps of Repair by Connective Tissue

A. *Development of Granulation Tissue*

There is proliferation of fibroblasts and endothelial cells within 3–5 days. Granulation tissue appears as pink, soft and granular.

B. *Connective Tissue Deposition*

Deposition occurs in four steps.

1. *Angiogenesis*

Development of new blood vessels from pre-existing blood vessels is known as neovascularization. It occurs as follows
- Proteolytic degradation of basement of parent vessel
- Migration of endothelial cells towards angiogenic stimulus
- Proliferation of endothelial cells
- Maturation of endothelial cells(remodeling) by inhibition of growth
- Recruitment of parietal cells. Angiogenesis increases vascular permeability which leads to increased deposition of plasma proteins in extracellular matrix.

2. *Fibrosis*

Within framework of granulation tissue migration and proliferation of fibroblast occur. Fibroblast migrates in extracellular matrix by factors like TGFB, PDGF, EGF, FGF, fibrogenic cytokines, IL-1, TNF-α.

3. *Extracellular Matrix Deposition*

Endothelial cells and fibroblast decrease in number and extracellular matrix deposition increases with time. The process is controlled by same factors as for fibroblastic proliferation. Highly vascular granulation scaffolding is converted into avascular scar tissue.

4. *Tissue Remodeling*

Growth factors stimulate collagen synthesis and also synthesize enzymes to degrade extracellular matrix. Remodeling takes place with the help of metalloproteinase like interstitial collagenase, gelatinase, stromalysins, MBMM. These are inhibited by tissue inhibitors of metalloproteinase.

Complications of Wound Repair

- Deficient scar formation because of inadequate granulation tissue leads to wound dehiscence and ulceration
- Excessive formation of repair component leads to keloid/hypertrophied scar, exuberant granulation tissue, fibromatosis
- Contracture deformity develops due to stretching by scar tissue
- Fibrosis associated with chronic inflammatory disease leads to disabling disease For example, rheumatoid arthritis, lung fibrosis and cirrhosis.

6

Cellular Adaptations

DEFINITION

Cellular adaptations are adjustments made at cellular level in response to stress by the body with an object,

- To meet out physiological need (Physiological adaptation)
- To survive in non-lethal pathologic conditions (Pathological adaptation)

Cellular adaptations may revert back if stimulus is withdrawn. If stimulating factor persist for long duration cell undergo irreversible injury (death) or progress further to neoplastic transformation.

Cellular changes may be

A. Decrease or increase in size (atrophy/hypertrophy)
B. Change in differentiations (metaplasia/dysplasia)

ATROPHY

Reduction in number and size of parenchymal cells of an organ or part which was once normal is called atrophy. It is different from hypoplasia/aplasia, in which the organ or tissue is small/absent since birth because of developmental defect (Fig. 6.1).

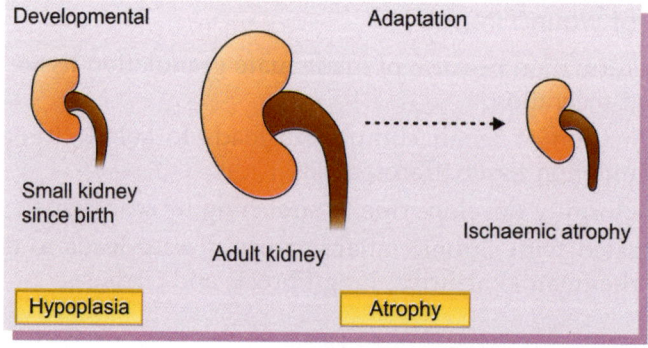

Fig. 6.1: Difference between hypoplasia and atrophy

Physiologic Causes of Atrophy (As the result of normal process of aging)
- Atrophy of lymphoid tissue in lymph node, appendix, thymus
- Atrophy of gonads after menopause (loss of endocrinal stimulation)
- Atrophy of brain (atherosclerosis)

Pathological Causes

1. Starvation

Depletion of carbohydrate, exhausted fat store and then protein catabolism leads to general weakness, followed by emaciation and ultimately cachaxia supervene. For example, carcinoma patients, severely ill patients.

2. Ischaemia

Gradual diminution of blood supply due to any reason decreases the cell mass and leads to atrophy of the organ.

For example, atrophic kidneys due to renal artery stenosis, brain atrophy due to atherosclerosis.

3. Disuse

Prolong diminution of functional activity results in shrinkage of the part or organ. For example, wasting of muscles of limb occurs, if a limb is immobilized in the cast because of fracture. Atrophy of pancreas in obstruction of pancreatic duct.

4. Neuropathic

Nerve stimulation is required to make the tissue vital. If neural transmission is interrupted because of any reason, it leads to wasting of that muscle. For example, wasting of muscles in poliomyelitis, or motor neuron disease

5. Endocrine

Loss of endocrine regulatory mechanism results in decreased metabolic activity of that particular gland or organ. If stimulating hormone is low for long duration, it results in reduced size of gland/organ. For example, hypopituitarism leads to atrophy of thyroid gland, adrenal gland, and gonads.

6. Pressure

Prolong pressure from tumor/cyst cause compression atrophy of the organ. For example, erosion of spine by tumor in nerve root. Erosion of skull by meningioma, Erosion of sternum by aneurysm of aorta.

7. Idiopathic

No obvious cause. For example, myopathies, testicular atrophy. Morphologic changes in atrophy.

Gross Features

- Organ is small and shrunken

Microscopic Features

- Cells are reduced in size due to
  - Decrease in mitochondria
  - Decrease in microfilaments
  - Decrease in endoplasmic reticulum
  - Increase in number of autophagic vacuoles, so that lipofuscin pigments are formed (known as Brown atrophy)

HYPERTROPHY

Definition

It is characterized by increase in size of parenchymal cells resulting in enlargement of the organ/tissue. Cell number is not increased. For example, cardiac muscles get hypertrophied to meet out physiological need. Usually nondividing cells undergo hypertrophy without hyperplasia.

Physiological Causes of Hypertrophy and Hyperplasia

- Increase in size of uterus during pregnancy
- Hypertrophy of breast during lactation

Pathological Causes of Hypertrophy

1. Cardiac left ventricular hypertrophy because of systemic hypertension, aortic valve disease, and mitral insufficiency.
2. Hypertrophy of smooth muscles:
   - Of stomach in pyloric stenosis
   - Of intestine in strictures
   - Of muscular arteries in hypertension
3. Skeletal muscles hypertrophy in athletes, manual laborers.
4. Compensatory hypertrophy of contralateral kidney if one kidney is removed or damaged.

Morphological Changes

Gross Features

Organ is enlarged and become heavy due to hypertrophy.

Microscopic Features

Enlargement in size of muscle fibers is seen because of increased synthesis of DNA, RNA, and organelles (mitochondria, endoplasmic reticulum).

HYPERPLASIA

Definition

It is characterized by increase in number of parenchymal cells, often occurs with hypertrophy.

It is because of increase recruitment of cells from G_0 phase of cell cycle to undergo mitosis. Following cells can undergo hyperplasia

- Labile cells (skin, mucous membrane epithelial cells, bone marrow cells)
- Stable cells (liver, pancreas, kidney, adrenal, thyroid)

Permanent cells (neuron, cardiac, skeletal muscles) have little or no capacity for hyperplasia. Compare it from neoplasia, which shows loss of growth regulatory mechanism (i.e. growth persist irrespective of stimulus). In hyperplasia growth persists as long as stimulus is present.

Physiological Causes of Hyperplasia

1. *Hormonal*

Under the influence of hormone stimulus hyperplasia tales place. For example

- Breast hyperplasia in female at puberty, pregnancy, lactation
- Uterine hyperplasia in pregnancy
- Endometrial proliferation in proliferative phase of menstrual cycle
- Prostatic hyperplasia in old age

2. *Compensatory*

For example

- Regeneration of liver in partial removal of liver tissue or traumatic injury
- Regeneration of skin after abrasion

Pathological Causes

- Endometrial hyperplasia due to excessive estrogenic stimulation
- Skin wart formation occurs due to hyperplasia of epidermal layers because of papilloma virus
- Formation of granulation tissue in wound healing

Morphological Changes

Gross features: There is enlargement of affected organ/tissue.
Microscopic features: Increased rate of DNA synthesis and increased cell division.

METAPLASIA

Metaplasia is the transformation of one type of cell to another in response to abnormal stimuli which often reverts back on removal of stimulus. If stimulus persists metaplastic cells may transform into carcinoma.

Types

1. Squamous Epithelial Metaplasia

It occurs due to chronic irritations (mechanical, chemical, and infective). For example,

- Pseudostratified ciliated columnar epithelial lining of bronchus is converted into squamous epithelial lining is patients of chronic cigarette smokers
- Endocervical columnar epithelium is changed to squamous epithelium in prolapse of uterus
- Columnar epithelium of gall bladder undergo squamous metaplasia in response to mechanical trauma due calculus in cholilithiasis.
- Squamous metaplasia is seen in prostate in chronic prostatitis and estrogen therapy
- Vitamin A deficiency leads to squamous metaplasia of nasal, bronchial, lacrimal and salivary gland epithelium

2. Columnar Epithelial Metaplasia

For example

- Intestinal metaplasia seen in chronic healed gastric ulcer
- In cervical erosion squamous epithelium is changed into columnar epithelium.

3. Mesenchymal Osseous Metaplasia

Mesenchymal osseous metaplasia is the formation of bone in fibrous/cartilage and myxoid tissue. For example

- Mönckeberg's medical calcific sclerosis of blood vessels in old age
- Myositis ossificans (osseous calcification in muscle tissue)
- Cartilage of larynx and bronchi in elderly undergo osseous metaplasia

4. Mesenchymal Cartilaginous Metaplasia

Mesenchymal cartilaginous metaplasia is the formation of cartilage in fibrous, bone or myxoid tissue. For example

   During healing of fractures when there is undue mobility of fractured part, healed part does not get ossified and soft cartilaginous tissue persist.

DYSPLASIA

It is characterized by disordered cellular proliferation often accompanied with metaplasia and hyperplasia. Dysplasia is seen in epithelial cells only. Dysplasia can be designated as atypical hyperplasia (Fig. 6.2).

Cytological Changes

- Hyperplasia of epithelial layers
- Loss of polarity
- Anisocytosis, anisonucleosis
- Increase nuclear/cytoplasmic ratio

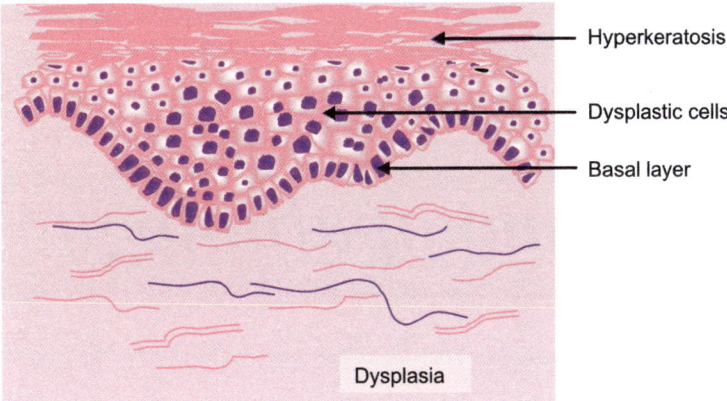

Fig. 6.2: Dysplasia

- Hyperchromatism
- Increased numbers of mitoses

For example
- Uterine cervical dysplasia
- Respiratory epithelial dysplasia

Dysplasia may progress to carcinoma *in situ*, and then into invasive carcinoma if the stimulating factor persist. Carcinoma *in situ* is cancer confined to the epithelial layers only. When there is invasion into the stroma, it is overt carcinoma.

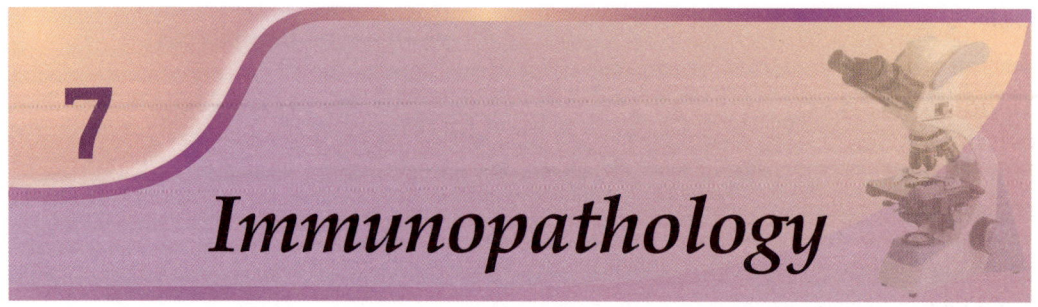

Immunopathology

IMMUNE SYSTEM

Immune system consists of:

Antigen

It is a proteinaceous substance which can stimulate antibody production.

Hepten

It is a nonproteinaceous substance, when it combines with a protein, it can stimulate antibody production.

Antibody

These are produced in response to antigen stimulus. These are immunoglobulin of five types: IgG, IgA, IgM, IgE, and IgD.

Classification of Immunity

A. On the Basis of their Action

- Humoral (mediated through antibodies)
- Cellular (mediated through neutrophils, macrophages and natural killer cells)

B. On the Basis of Specificity

1. **Innate** present since birth (without antigen specificity, it forms 1st line of defense)
   - Humoral is through complement
   - Cellular is through lymphocytes, macrophages, and natural killer cell (NK cells)
2. **Acquired** later on in the life (specific for an antigen)
   - Humoral is through antibodies formed by B lymphocytes
   - Cellular is through T lymphocytes

Cells of Immune System

1. T Lymphocytes

Thymus derived cells which mediate cellular immunity resides in Para cortical region of lymph nodes and periarteriolar sheath of spleen and constitute 60–70% of circulating lymphocytes. T lymphocytes can recognize cell bound antigens by their specific T cell receptors. They express CD-3 proteins.

About 60% mature cells also express CD-4 and 30% express CD-8 proteins. Rest 10% express CD-2, CD-11, CD-28 and CD-40

- CD-4+T lymphocytes (helper cells) constitute 60% of T mature lymphocytes and produce cytokines which help to B cells in producing antibodies and macrophages in destruction of phagocytosed microbes.
- CD-8+T lymphocytes constitute 30% of mature lymphocytes (CD-4 to CD-8 ratio is 2:1). It act as cytotoxic cells and directly kills virus infected cells or tumor cell.

2. B Lymphocytes

Bone marrow derived lymphocytes which mediate humoral immunity are found in cortex of lymph node, white pulp of spleen, tonsils, lymphoid tissue of GIT. They constitute 10–20% of circulating lymphocytes. When activated they differentiate into plasma cells, which synthesize antibodies and memory B cells. Memory B cells can recognize antigen later on when exposed to same antigen.

3. Dendritic Cells

These cells bear branched projection hence the name. They process antigen material and present to other cells of immune system. These are of two types:

- **Interdigitating dendritic cells** are nonphagocytic cells and are present in the skin (Langerhans cells), inner lining of nose, lung, stomach and intestine.
- **Follicular dendritic cells** are located in germinal centers of lymphoid follicles and spleen. They augment secondary antibody response.

4. Macrophages

These cells process and present antigens to immunocompetent T cells and are effecter cells in delayed hypersensitivity and humoral immunity.

5. Natural Killer Cells (NK cells)

These are large granular lymphocytes, constitute 10–15% of circulating lymphocytes and secrete TNF, IFN, and GMCSF.

HLA SYSTEM

HLA system regulate immune system. Genes regulating HLA are located over chromosomes number 6 are known as major histocompatibility complex (MHC or HLA complex). MHC present over chromosome no. 6 decides the molecule to be formed over surface of cells which bind to foreign peptide or prevent their binding.

Classification of HLA System

1. Class I antigen—HLA-A, HLA-B, HLA-C are located on all nucleated cells of body.
2. Class II antigen—HLA-D are found on macrophages and B and T lymphocytes.
3. Class III antigen—These are located on components of complement system.

Role and Significance of HLA System

1. Organ transplantation
2. Regulation of immune system
    i. Class I regulate functions of CD-8 (cytotoxic) cells
    ii. Class II regulates functions of CD-4 (helper) cells
3. Association of disease with HLA. For example, ankylosing spondilitis is associated with HLA-B27. Rheumatoid arthritis and diabetes mellitus are associated with HLA-DR4

ACQUIRED IMMUNODEFICIENCY SYNDROME (AIDS)

It was recognized in 1981 in USA.

Etiology

Human immunodeficiency virus (HIV). Retrovirus HIV is a type of HTLV (Human T lymphoma/leukemia virus). CD-4 molecules on T lymphocytes are the target of attack leading to cytolysis.

Structure of HIV (Fig 7.1)

Routes of Transmission

1. Sexual Contact

    i. Homosexual/bisexual in USA
    ii. Heterosexual in Africa/Asia

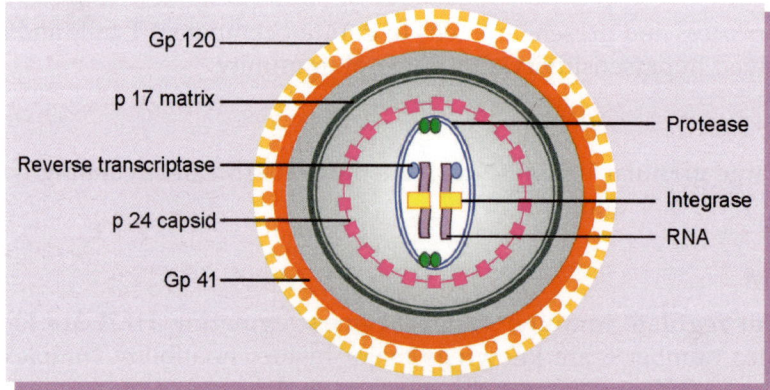

Fig. 7.1: Schematic diagram of HIV virion

2. *Parental*

   i. Intravenous drug users

  ii. Hemophilic receiving regular blood transfusion

 iii. Recipients of blood and blood products

3. *Perinatal*

From mother to newborn through placenta

Pathogenesis (Fig. 7.2)

1. *T lymphocytes*

CD4+molecule is a high affinity receptor of HIV.

- Gp 120 of HIV binds to CD-4+molecule and conformational changes in gp 120 creating a new recognition site
- Fusion peptide present at gp 41 is inserted in to the cell membrane and viral genome enters inside the cell
- After internalization, viral genome undergoes reverse transcription to form DNA which is integrated into host genome and viral particles are synthesized
- Synthesized viral particles are released after cell lysis

2. *Monocytes and Macrophages*

When person is infected, the monocytes and macrophages do not show cytopathic effect, they act as reservoir for HIV infection and provide site for viral replication in late phase of disease.

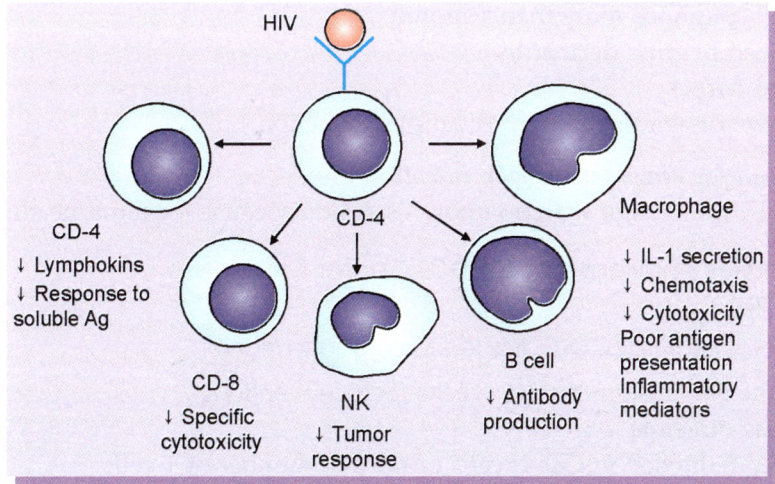

Fig. 7.2: Pathogenesis of HIV infection

3. Nervous System

Infected monocytes are carried to central nervous system. It infects the macrophages and glial cells. Neurons are not infected. Lesions produced are
- Acute aseptic meningitis
- Subacute encephalitis
- Vacuolar myelopathy
- Peripheral neuropathy

4. B lymphocytes

Derangement of B cell function occurs. Decreased immunoglobulin and increased γ-globulin leads to immune complex formation.

5. Dendritic Cells

Virus reach to regional lymph nodes and follicular dendritic cells get infected. It acts as reservoir.

Clinical Features

Major Signs

- Weight loss more than 10% of body weight
- Chronic diarrhea for more than 1 month
- Prolong fever for more than 1 month

Minor Signs

- Recurrent oropharyngeal candidiasis
- Persistent generalized lymphadenopathy
- Persistent cough for more than 1 month
- Generalized pruritic dermatitis
- Recurrent herpes
- Progressive disseminated herpes simplex infection

WHO criteria for diagnosis of HIV infection are
2 major and 1 minor sign with no known secondary cause for immune suppression

Clinical Phases of Disease and CDC (Center for disease control) Classification

A. Early Acute Phase (CDC grade I, acute infection)

1. Immune responses after 3–6 weeks (Seroconversion)
2. Increase viraemia
3. Marked reduction in CD-4+cells or normal number of T cells
4. Rise in CD-8+cells
5. Nonspecific viral illness

B. *Middle Chronic Phase* (CDC grade II—asymptomatic infection)

(Grade III—persistent generalized lymphadenopathy)

- Latent stage may be up to 10 years
- Viraemia increases
- CD-4+ cell decreases
- CD-8+ cells increases

C. *Crisis Phase* (CDC grade IV)

- Marked viraemia
- CD4+ cells decreases below 200/cu mm
- Constitutional disease   (CDC Subgroup A)
- Neurological disease   (CDC Subgroup B)
- Secondary opportunistic infection   (CDC Subgroup C)
- Secondary neoplasm   (CDC Subgroup D)
- Other conditions   (CDC Subgroup E)

Pathological Changes

1. Opportunistic infections
2. Bacterial, fungal, viral, protozoal and helminthic infection
3. AIDS associated cancers
4. Kaposi's sarcoma, B cell non-Hodgkin's lymphoma
5. Hematological manifestations
6. Nephropathy
7. Focal segmental glomerulosclerosis
8. Lymphoid tissue
9. Follicular hyperplasia to involution and finally atrophic lymph nodes

Laboratory Diagnosis

Specific Tests

1. Serological tests
   i. In acute illness—ELISA test for antigen detection (p24)
   ii. Asymptomatic patient—ELISA test for antibody detection
2. Western blot test (more specific)
3. Immunofluorescent test
4. Antigen detection by recombinant DNA technique
5. Viral isolation and culture
6. PCR New gold standard test in all stages of HIV

Nonspecific Test

1. CD-4 and CD-8 counts

2. Lymphopenia
3. Lymph node biopsy
4. Thrombocytopenia
5. Increased β-microglobulin level

HYPERSENSITIVITY REACTIONS

Exaggerated immune response to an antigen is called hypersensitivity reactions. Symptoms may be from simple itching to fatal state. Immunity confers resistance offered to infection, while hypersensitivity denotes allergy.

Classification

Depending upon rapidity and duration of immune response:

Immediate type	Delayed type
• Reaction occurs with in seconds	• Reaction occurs in 24 to 48 hours
• Mediated by humoral antibodies	• Mediated by cellular response
• It may be of Type I, II or III	• Classified as Type IV

Type I Hypersensitivity (Anaphylactic/Atopic Hypersensitivity)

It is characterized by rapid response to antigen in previously sensitized individual, mediated by IgE antibodies. IgE stimulates basophils in blood and mast cells in tissue and releases (Fig. 7.3)

Anaphylactic Mediators (Anaphylotoxins) like

1. Vasoactive amines
   • Histamine
   • 5-hydroxytryptaphan
2. AA metabolites
   • Chemotactic factors for neutrophils and eosinophils
   • Prostaglandin
   • Thromboxane
3. Platelet activating factors

Effects produced are:
• Increased vascular permeability
• Increased gastric, nasal and lacrimal secretions
• Vasoconstriction followed by vasodilatation
• Smooth muscle contraction
• Low blood pressure leading to shock

Examples of anaphylaxis are:
Systemic anaphylaxis caused by
• Administration of antiserum

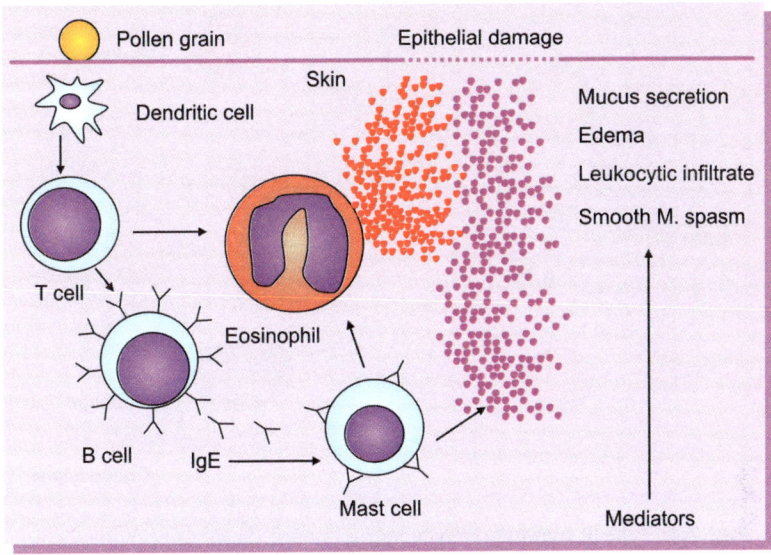

Fig. 7.3: Pathogenesis of Type I

- Administration of certain drugs like penicillin
- Bee sting

Symptoms produced are:
Itching, erythema, dyspnoea, diarrhoea, shock, may be fatal if severe
Local anaphylaxis caused by
- Hay fever/seasonal allergic rhinitis due to pollen grains
- Bronchial asthma due to allergen like house dust
- Food allergy due to ingestion of certain food like fish, cow milk
- Urticaria (cutaneous anaphylaxis)
- Angioedema (edema of lip, tongue and eyelids)

Type II Hypersensitivity (Cytotoxic reactions)

Hypersensitivity reaction which cause injury to the cell with the help of antibodies. Depending on the mechanism involved it is of three types:
1. Cytotoxic antibodies to blood cells
2. Cytotoxic antibody to cell component
3. Antibody dependent cell mediated cytotoxicity

1. Cytotoxic Antibody to Blood Cell (Complement dependent)

It involves two mechanisms (Fig. 7.4)
- Blood cells surface antigens combine with IgG/IgM antibodies and activate complement and direct causing lysis of cells by membrane attack complex

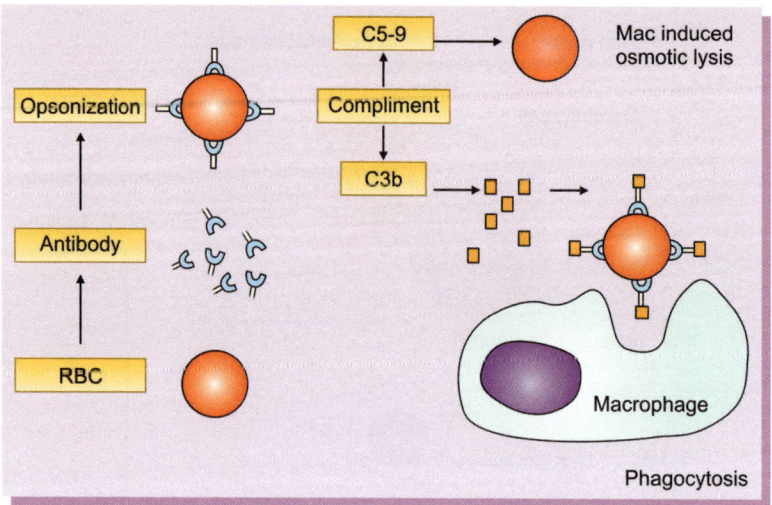

Fig. 7.4: Type II hypersensitivity, complement dependent cytotoxicity

• Opsonization of blood cells by C3b and C4b and destruction by phagocytosis
  For example, autoimmune haemolytic anaemia, transfusion reactions, erythroblastosis foetalis, idiopathic thrombocytopenia.

2. Cytotoxic Antibody to Cell Component

Auto antibodies developed against cellular component cause injury to cell. For example
• In Graves' disease, thyroid receptor antibodies cause hyperthyroidism
• In myasthenia gravis, antibodies to acetylcholine receptor cause muscular weakness
• Antisperm antibodies results in motility impairment of sperms

3. Antibody Dependent Cell Mediated Cytotoxicity (ADCC)

Antibodies bind to target cells. Fc fragment of antibody is recognized by phagocytic cells causing lysis of target cell. For example, tumor cells and parasitic destruction.

Type III Hypersensitivity (Immune complex reactions) (Fig. 7.5)

Deposition of antigen-antibody complexes leads to activation of complement which leads to tissue damage. Agents who induce the reaction are:
• Exogenous agents like infectious agents, drugs and chemicals
• Endogenous agents like tumor antigen, nuclear antigen, immunoglobulin

Immune complex reactions are of two types:
1. Local reaction (Arthus reaction)
2. Systemic reaction (serum sickness)

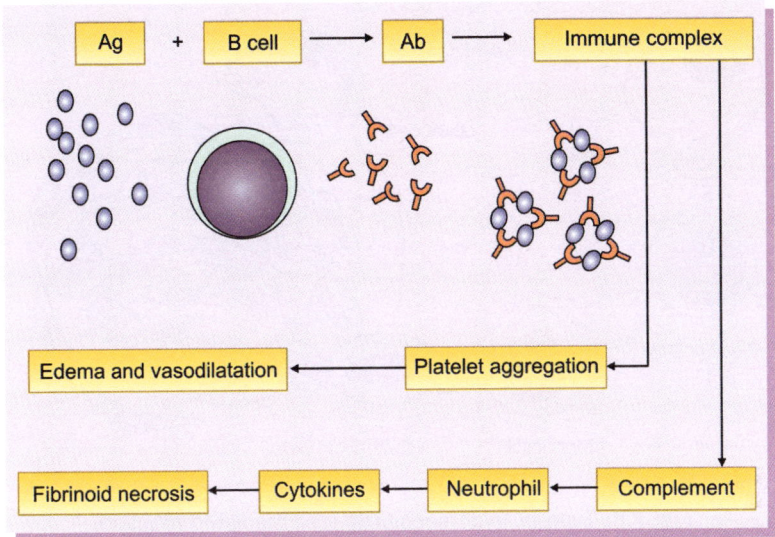

Fig. 7.5: Immune complex deposition (Type III hypersensitivity reaction)

1. Local Reaction (Arthus reaction)

It is defined as localized tissue necrosis of skin resulting from acute immune complex vasculitis involving complement fixing antibodies. Large immune complexes are precipitated in blood vessel wall. For example, intradermal antitetanus serum leads to fibrinoid necrosis (vasculitis). It is presented as edema, haemorrhage and ulceration in few hours with peak in 4–10 hours.

2. Systemic Reaction (Serum sickness)

Antigen and Antibody complexes are deposited at exposed basement membrane of glomerulus, lungs, choroid plexus, uveal tract and synovium. They activate complement resulting in release of vasoactive amines, chemotactic factors and anaphylatoxins. For example, post streptococcal glomerulonephritis, collagen vascular disease like systemic lupus erythematosus (SLE), poly arteritis nodosa (PAN), rheumatoid arthritis, Goodpasture's syndrome, arthritis.

Type IV Hypersensitivity (Cell mediated reaction)

A. Classical Delayed Hypersensitivity (Fig. 7.6)

It is mediated through sensitized CD-4+cells. For example
- Tuberculin reaction (Mantoux test)
- When intradermal PPD (purified protein derivative) is given to previously sensitized person, an erythema and induration appear at the site of injection after 8–12 hours and peaks at 24 to 72 hours.
- Tubercular granulomatous inflammation
- Tuberculoid leprosy

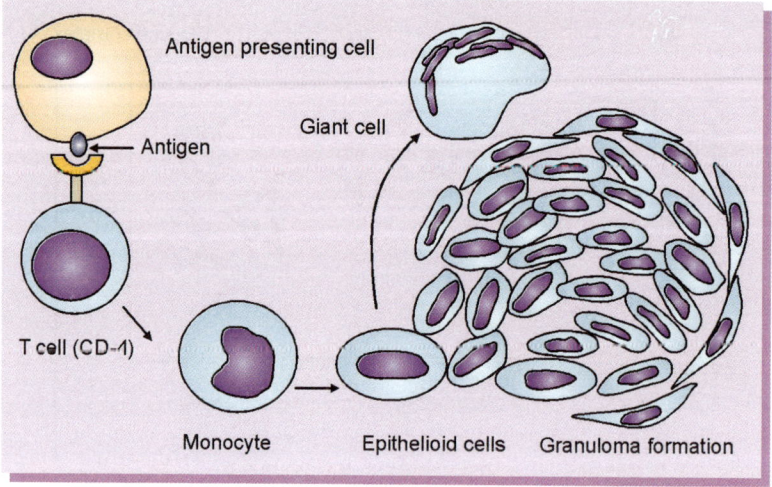

Fig. 7.6: Type IV hypersensitivity (cell mediated reaction)

B. *T cell mediated Cytotoxicity*

Sensitized CD-8+T lymphocytes cause lysis of cells bearing antigen. For example
- Virus infected cells
- Tumor cell lysis
- Incompatible transplanted tissue (graft rejection)

AUTOIMMUNE DISEASES

Since foetal life a person has ability to recognize self antigen and hence B lymphocyte and T lymphocytes do not react. This phenomenon is called immune tolerance.

When there is loss of this kind of tolerance, immune system of body react with self antigen and produce symptoms. Such diseases which are produced because of loss of immunological tolerance are known as autoimmune diseases.

Autoimmunity is a state of immune system which fails to recognize difference between self and foreign antigens.

Pathogenesis

Exact mechanism involved is not clear, however, three factors has been recognized.
1. Immunological factor—Failure of immunological tolerance due to
    - Polyclonal activation of B lymphocytes by stimulus which bypass the T cell immunological tolerance.
    - Generation of self reacting B lymphocyte clone which bypass T cell tolerance.
    - Decreased T suppressor activity and increased T helper activity.
    - Failure of mechanism of tolerance by interference with anti idiotypic network.
    - Release of sequestrated antigen to immune system.

2. Genetic factor—Increased expression of class II HLA antigens and familial clustering has been observed in autoimmune diseases, suggestive of genetic factors responsible for autoimmunity.
3. Microbial factors—Infections with viruses, for example, EBV, bacteria like streptococci, *Klebsiella* and *Mycoplasma* has been found to be associated with autoimmune diseases.

Classification

Depending upon type of autoantibody, autoimmune diseases have been classified into two types:
1. Organ specific autoimmune diseases like Hashimoto's thyroiditis, Graves' disease, ulcerative colitis, Crohn's disease, myasthenia gravis, etc.
2. Non-organ specific autoimmune diseases like systemic lupus erythematosus (SLE), rheumatoid arthritis, polyarteritis nodosa (PAN), Sjögren's syndrome, etc.

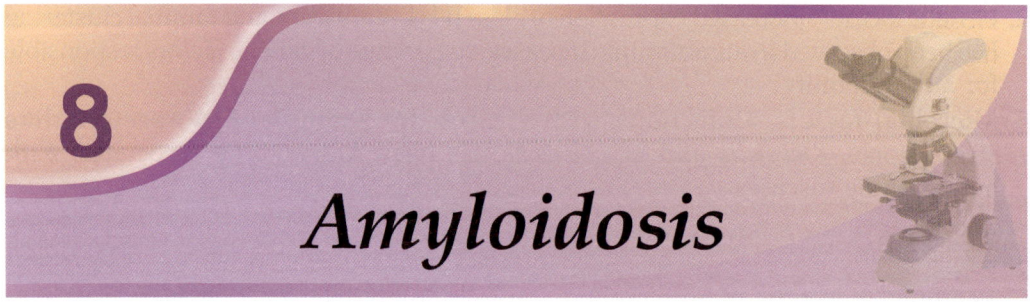

8

Amyloidosis

DEFINITION

Amyloidosis is a group of diseases characterized by deposition of fibrillar proteinaceous substance in extracellular matrix.

Rokitansky (1842) first described the Amyloidosis. "Amyloid" name was given by Virchow; because amyloid material has resemblance with starch (amyl means starch). The characteristic reaction of starch, i.e. violet color by iodine and brown by sulphuric acid was shown by amyloid material. However, now it is clear that amyloid material is proteinaceous in nature hence now an alternate term "β Fibrillosis" has been given because of its β pleated fibrillar protein composition.

Physical Nature of Amyloid Material

- It consists of fibrils, which are delicate non-branching filaments of indefinite length

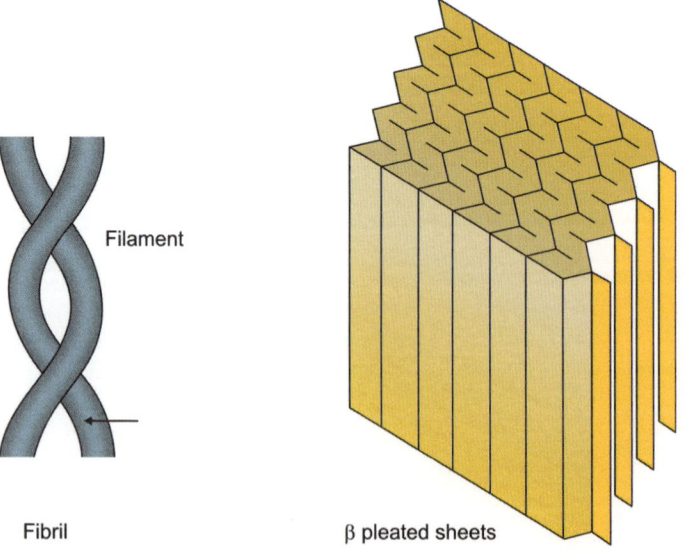

Filament

Fibril   β pleated sheets

Fig. 8.1: Physical structure of amyloid

- Fibril is made up of 1–4 aligned aggregates (7.5–10 nm diameters) of proto fibrils (filament), which are arranged in cross β pleated pattern (Fig. 8.1)

Chemical Nature of Amyloid Material

It is an extracellular, homogenous, hyaline, eosinophilic, amorphous, proteinaceous material composed of two proteins
1. Fibril protein (90%)
2. P component (10%)

1. Fibril Protein

Two major forms of fibril protein and one group of heterogeneous fibril proteins have been identified
A. Amyloid light chain (AL) protein
B. Amyloid associated (AA) protein
C. Other amyloid like protein

A. AL Protein

- These are polypeptide chain made up of light chain of immunoglobulin (Kappa and Lambda chain) produced by plasma cells
- These are seen in plasma cell dyscrasia like multiple myeloma and Waldenström's macroglobulinaemia

B. AA Proteins

- AA proteins are polypeptide chain having 78 amino acids
- These are derived from serum amyloid associated protein (SAA) which is an acute phase reactant in serum bound to HDL3 lipoprotein
- It is synthesized in liver and seen in inflammatory conditions (secondary amyloidosis.

C. Other Amyloid Protein

- ATTR (amyloid transthyretin).
  It is protein which transport thyroxin and retinal protein. Its mutant form is deposited in familial amyloidosis.
- $β_2$-microglobulin is associated with long-term haemodialysis.
- A β amyloid protein is deposited in Alzheimer's disease. It is derived from its precursor protein.
- Hormone precursor (procalcitonin, proinsulin)
  These are deposited as amyloid material.

2. P Component

It has non fibrillar pentagonal profile, synthesized in liver. It is readily soluble glycoprotein, resembling to α-glycoprotein of serum and related to CRP.

Pathogenesis

Amyloidosis is not a single disease and different mechanisms are involved in different forms.

1. Abnormal amount of normal proteins, which are unstable, forms oligomers and fibrils. For example

AL Protein Deposition

- In immunoglobulin synthesis disorder (monoclonal gammopathy) large amount of immunoglobulins are synthesized
- Immunoglobulins undergo partial degradation (limited proteolysis) in macrophages
- P component and glycosaminoglycans play some unknown role in amyloid deposition

AA Amyloid Deposition

- Chronic inflammation cause long-term destruction
- Macrophages activation results in increased IL-1 an IL-6 level
- Amyloid enhancing factors (AEF) leads to AA amyloid deposition

2. Normal amount of mutant unstable proteins are synthesized, which get aggregated. For example, deposition of transthyretin as ATTR protein.

Classification

A. Systemic (generalized)
   1. Primary amyloidosis
   2. Secondary amyloidosis
   3. Haemodialysis associated amyloidosis
   4. Heredofamilial amyloidosis
B. Localized
   1. Senile cardiac amyloidosis
   2. Senile cerebral amyloidosis
   3. Endocrine amyloidosis

A. Systemic Amyloidosis

1. Primary Amyloidosis

- Protein deposited is AL type
- 30% cases are seen in plasma cell dyscrasia
- 70% cases are idiopathic
- Organs involved are heart, bowel, skin, and skeletal muscle.

2. Secondary Amyloidosis

Protein deposited is AA type. It is seen in

- Chronic infective conditions like tuberculosis, bronchiectasis, chronic osteomyelitis, leprosy

- Inflammatory diseases like ulcerative colitis, Crohn's disease
- Tumors like renal cell carcinoma, Hodgkin's disease
  Organs involved are liver, spleen, and kidney

3. Haemodialysis Associated Amyloidosis

Long-term (>10 years) dialysis in chronic renal failure leads to deposition of β_2-microglobulin in synovium, joints, tendon sheath.

4. Heredofamilial Amyloidosis

Theses are rare type amyloidosis.
A. *Familial Mediterranean fever (Fever and serositis):* It has autosomal recessive inheritance. AA type proteins are deposited in solid abdominal organs
B. *Hereditary polyneuropathic amyloidosis:* It has autosomal dominant inheritance. Protein deposited is transthyretin and organs involved are peripheral and autonomic nerves.

B. Localized Amyloidosis

1. Senile Cardiac Amyloidosis

Fifty percent people of >70 years of age shows amyloid deposition in heart and aorta.

2. Senile Cerebral Amyloidosis

Sixty percent people of Alzheimer's disease shows amyloid deposition in cerebral blood vessels.

3. Endocrine Amyloidosis

In medullary carcinoma of thyroid and islet tumor of pancreas amyloid deposited are derived from procalcitonin and proinsulin

Staining Characteristics of Amyloid Material

Stain	Color of amyloid material
Haemotoxylin and Eosin	Hyaline pink
Crystal violet (metachromatic stain)	Rose pink
Congo red	Orange in normal light
	Apple green birefringence in polarized light
Prior permanganate treatment + Congo red	Orange color suggest AL protein
	No orange color suggest AA protein
Fluorescent Thioflavin S	Yellow in UV light
Sulfated alcian blue	Blue green
PAS stain	Pink color

Morphological Features

1. Kidney is most common organ involved
   - Enlarged or normal in early stage and contracted in later stage

- Cut section shows pale waxy translucent appearance
- Glomerulus—Amyloid material deposition is seen on basement membrane and mesangial matrix. Luminal narrowing is evident due to basement membrane thickening. Distortion of capillary tuft is seen.
- Tubules—Amyloid deposition close to tubular epithelial basement membrane and inter tubular connective tissue are seen.
- Vessels—Lumen is narrowed.
2. Spleen, two patterns are seen
    A. Sago spleen
      - No marked splenomegaly
      - Cut surface shows translucent waxy nodules (sago grains)
      - Deposits of amyloid are seen in the walls of arterioles in white pulp, so that follicle is replaced by amyloid material
    B. Lardaceous spleen
      - Moderate to marked splenomegaly
      - Cut surface shows yellow map like areas (Lard means fat of pig which looks like map)
      - Deposits of amyloid material is seen in wall of splenic sinuses, small arterioles and connective tissue of red pulp, sparing white pulp.
3. Liver
    - Liver is enlarged, firm pale, and waxy
    - Amyloid deposits are seen the space of Disse
    - Later on it compresses the cord of hepatocytes
    - Finally atrophic hepatocytes are replaced by amyloid material
4. Heart
    - Size of heart appear normal or at times enlarged
    - Tiny amyloid deposits are seen underneath the endocardium and between myocardial fibers
5. Alimentary canal
    - Amyloid deposits can be seen at any level from mouth to anus
    - Amyloid deposits are seen around blood vessels
6. Tongue shows macroglossia
7. Others organs—Pituitary, thyroid, adrenals, skin, lymph nodes may be involved.

Diagnosis of Amyloidosis

Biopsy

- It requires demonstration of amyloid material in biopsy specimen or abdominal fat. Preferred organ for biopsy are kidneys, rectum, gingival.

Other Tests

- Serum electrophoresis
- Bone marrow aspiration smears examination

Prognosis is poor in generalized amyloidosis.

9

Haemodynamics

INTRODUCTION

Haemodynamic homeostasis is required to maintain the integrity of cell, tissue and organ. Haemodynamics includes osmotic pressure of plasma, hydrostatic pressure of flowing blood and blood vessels integrity.

Disturbances in haemodynamic homeostasis leads to many pathological states like

- Edema
- Congestion
- Haemorrhage
- Thrombosis
- Embolism
- Infarction
- Shock

EDEMA

Edema is defined as increased interstitial fluid in tissue and/or serous cavities.

For example, hydrothorax, pericardial effusion, peritoneal effusion. Generalized edema with subcutaneous swelling is called Anasarca.

Fluid balance in tissue across capillary is governed by

1. Capillary hydrostatic pressure (HP) which results in outward movement of fluid across endothelium.
2. Plasma colloid osmotic pressure (OP) which retains the fluid inside the capillaries.
3. Tissue oncotic pressure which retains the fluid in the tissue.
4. Hydrostatic pressure in tissue (tissue tension) which leads to outward flow of fluid from tissue.

Pressure difference between HP and OP in capillary (32–25 = 7 mmHg) produce driving force and leads to outward flow of plasma from capillaries at arterial end. At venous end of capillary inward force (25–12 = 13 mmHg) is created leading to uptake of plasma again into the capillaries. Small amount of fluid which is retained in tissue is drained through lymphatics. Such physiological pressure gradients maintain the fluid balance and integrity of tissue (Fig. 9.1).

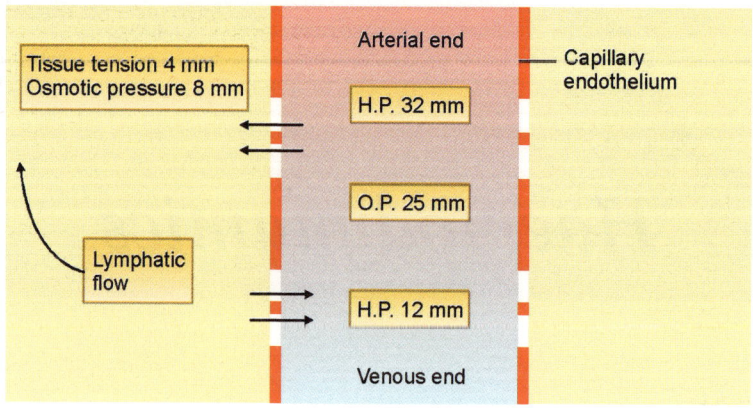

Fig. 9.1: Normal fluid balance

Pathophysiology of Edema

1. Increased Hydrostatic Pressure

Rise in hydrostatic pressure at venular end of capillary more than plasma oncotic pressure results in edema. For example, local impairment of venous flow in deep vein thrombosis, and generalized increase in venous pressure in congestive heart failure (Fig. 9.2).

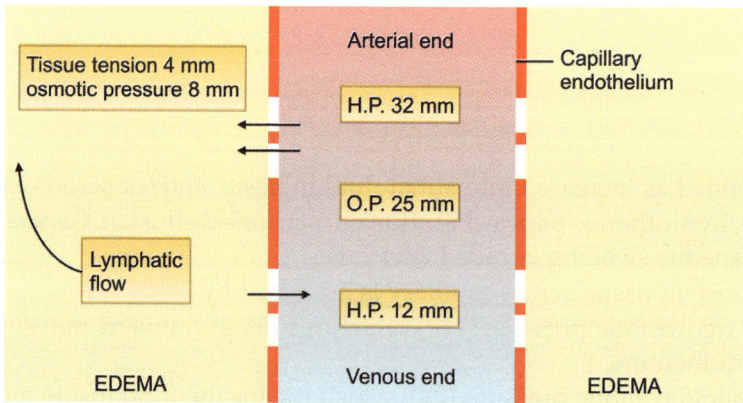

Fig. 9.2: Increased hydrostatic pressure

2. Reduced Plasma Oncotic Pressure

Reduced plasma oncotic pressure leads to non retention of fluid in capillaries resulting in increased flow of fluid in interstitium (Fig. 9.3). For example,

- In nephrotic syndrome, due to loss of albumin
- In cirrhosis, due to decreased synthesis of albumin
- In malnutrition, due to decreased protein in take
- Protein losing enteropathy, leads to increased loss of proteins

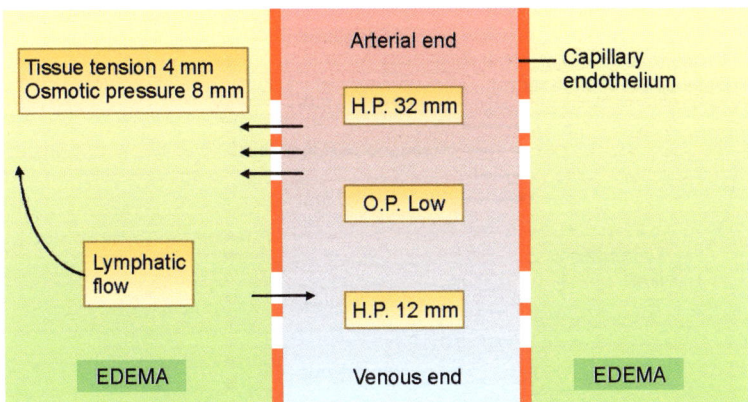

Fig. 9.3: Reduced plasma oncotic pressure

3. Lymphatic Obstruction

Obstruction to lymphatics causes accumulation of fluid in interstitium (Fig. 9.4). For example,
- In radical mastectomy, lymphoedema of arm develops
- Obstruction of thoracic duct by tumor, results in lymphoedema which when ruptures then it leads to development of chylothorax or chyloascites
- Inflammation of lymphatics by microfilariae leads to edema feet known as elephantiasis
- Mallory's disease, i.e. abnormal development of lymphatics leads to edema of the part affected

4. Increased Capillary Permeability

Injury caused by anoxia, drugs, and chemicals increases the capillary permeability (Fig. 9.5). For example
- Generalized edema in infections, poisoning, and allergic reaction
- Angioneurotic edema

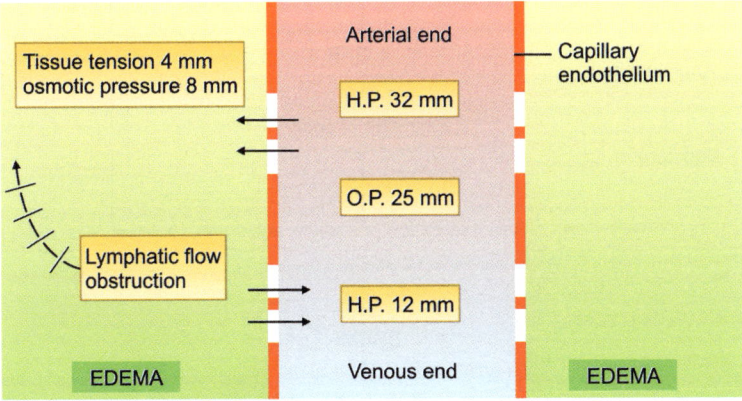

Fig. 9.4: Lymphatic obstruction

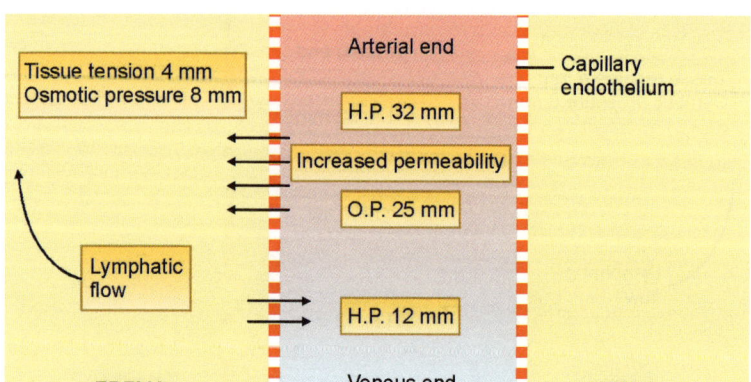

Fig. 9.5: Increased capillary permeability

5. *Sodium and Water Retention*

Sodium balance is maintained by
1. Intrinsic renal mechanism through glomerular filtration rate (GFR)
2. Extrinsic renal mechanism by renin—angiotensin—aldosterone mechanism.

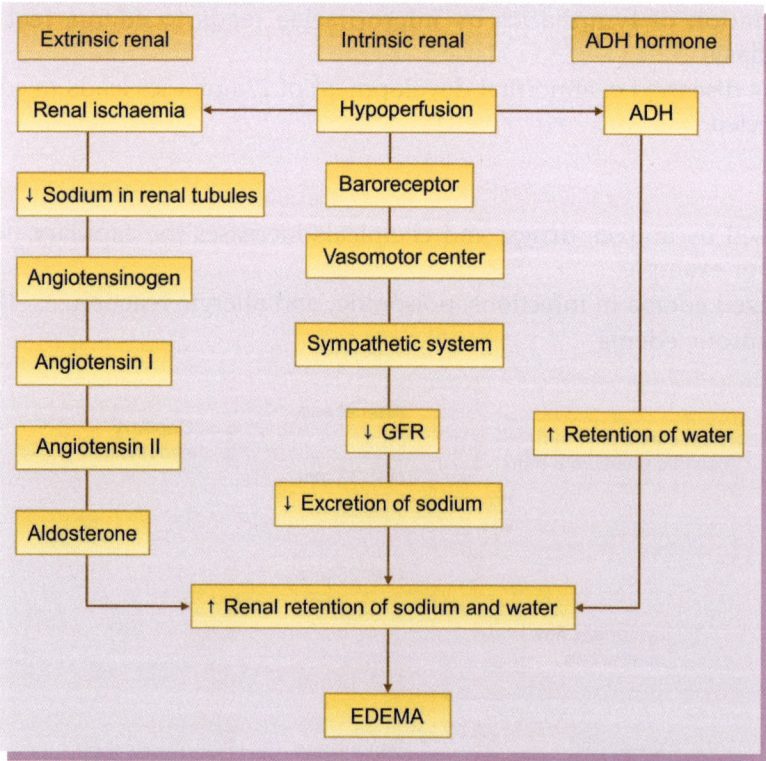

Fig. 9.6: Sodium and water retention

Sodium and water imbalance leads to edema, for example
- Excessive salt intake with renal disorder
- Increased tubular reabsorption of sodium
- Decreased renal perfusion
- Increased renin—angiotensin—aldosterone secretion

PATHOGENESIS OF RENAL EDEMA

Heavy proteinuria results in decreased oncotic pressure leading to generalized edema. Activation of renin angiotensin mechanism cause retention of sodium and water which further aggravate the condition (Fig. 9.7)

1. Nephrotic Syndrome

Gross features—Kidney are heavy with tense capsule
Microscopic features—Fluid separates connective tissue fibers

2. Glomerulonephritis (Nephritic edema)

It is due to increased reabsorption of sodium and water. Nephritic edema is milder as compared to nephrotic syndrome.

3. Acute Tubular Necrosis

It is because of shock and toxic chemicals. Tubular selective reabsorption capacity of tubule is lost resulting in increased reabsorption and oliguria.

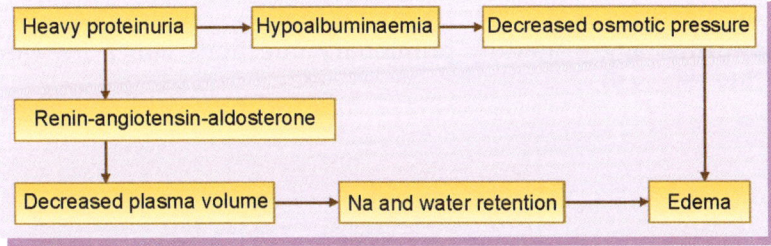

Fig. 9.7: Pathogenesis of renal edema

PATHOGENESIS OF CARDIAC EDEMA

In congestive heart failure generalized edema develops because of
1. Decreased output by heart results in sodium and water retention by aldosterone and ADH mechanisms. Decreased plasma volume cause decreased in GFR leading to more sodium and water retention.
2. Increased venous pressure and increased capillary hydrostatic pressure cause edema.
3. Chronic hypoxia due to CHF leads to tissue necrosis resulting in increased permeability of capillaries (Fig. 9.8).

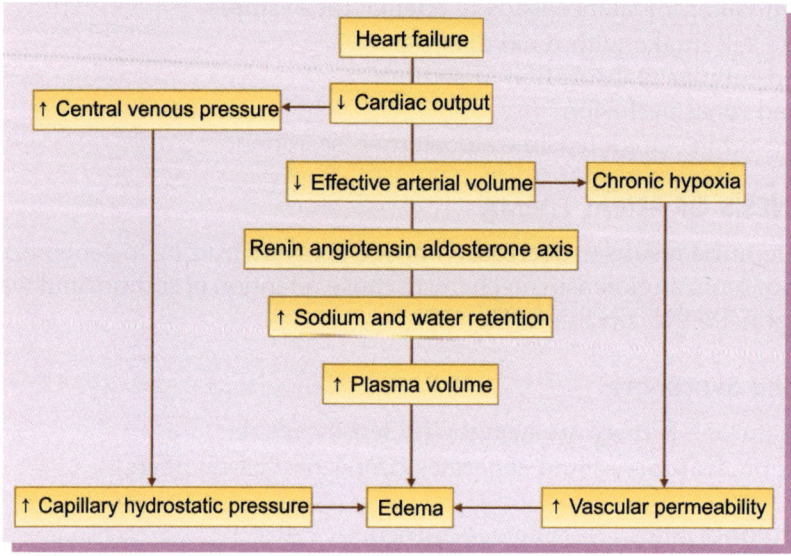

Fig. 9.8: Cardiac edema

PATHOGENESIS OF PULMONARY EDEMA

In left heart failure, mitral stenosis, pulmonary vein obstruction and pulmonary infections, pulmonary edema develops due to

- Increased pulmonary hydrostatic pressure in capillaries which leads to alveolar edema.
- Edema is further aggravated by pulmonary infections which increase capillary permeability (Fig. 9.9).

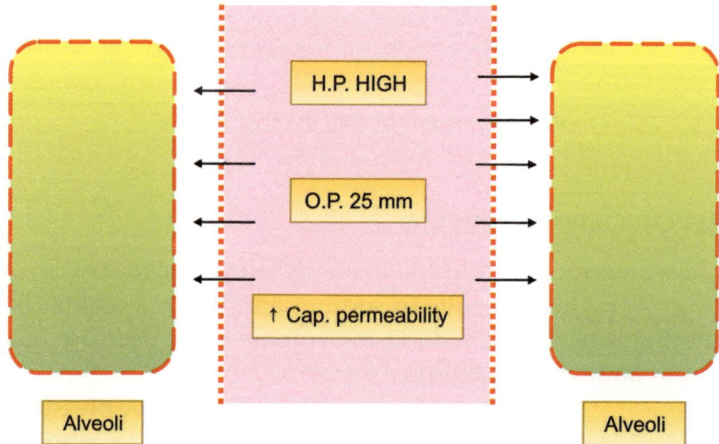

Fig. 9.9: Pulmonary edema

Morphological Features

- Lungs appear heavy and crepitant
- Fluid gets collected initially in interstitium and later on in alveoli. Chronic pulmonary edema leads to infection and chronic venous congestion. Lung appears brown (Brown induration)
- Widened alveolar septa with accumulation of haemosiderin laden macrophages (heart failure cells) are seen in alveoli

PATHOGENESIS OF CEREBRAL EDEMA

There are no lymphatics in brain.

1. Vasogenic edema develops because of increased capillary permeability.

   For example, contusion, infarction, abscess and tumors.
   - Brain becomes soft, swollen with flattened gyri and narrowed sulci
   - There is separation of tissue elements by edema fluid

2. Cytotoxic edema is due to defect in cellular osmoregulation. Blood brain barrier is intact. For example, acute hypoxia, toxins and metabolic derangements.
   - Fluid collection is intracellular. Cells become swollen and vacuolated

3. Interstitial edema leads to accumulation of excessive fluid in periventricular white matter crossing the ependymal lining.

   For example non-communicating hydrocephalus.

HYPEREMIA AND CONGESTION

Hyperemia: Increased volume of blood in dilated arterioles and capillaries of tissue of organ is termed as hyperemia.

Congestion: Congestion is collection of blood in capillary bed of tissue or organ due to impaired drainage.

Hyperemia	Congestion
• Local increase in blood volume in a dilated arteriole is hyperemia.	• Blood pooling due to impaired drainage is congestion.
• It is an active process.	• It is a passive process.
• Blood flow is augmented.	• Blood flow is impaired.
• Arteriolar dilatation is seen.	• Venous obstruction is seen.
• Tissue appears red due to oxygenated blood.	• Tissue appears blue-red due to deoxygenated blood.
• No edema is seen.	• Accompanied with edema.
For example: Fever, flushing, skeletal muscles during exercise	For example: Cardiac failure, local venous obstruction.

Types of Congestion

1. Acute or chronic (Fig. 9.10)
2. Systemic and local

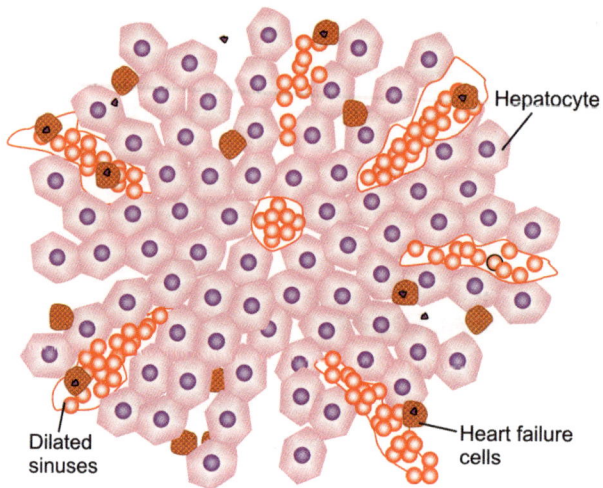

Hepatocyte

Dilated
sinuses

Heart failure
cells

Fig. 9.10: Chronic hepatic congestion

Morphological Changes in Congestion (Fig. 9.11)

1. Acute pulmonary congestion—Alveolar capillaries are engorged with blood. Alveolar septal edema/haemorrhage are seen.

2. Chronic pulmonary congestion (Brown induration). Long-standing venous congestion of lung due to left-sided heart failure leads to increased venous pressure and congestion
   • Heavy lungs firm in consistency
   • Cut surface is dark brown and frothy blood oozes on pressure
   • Thickened fibrotic septa, dilated septal capillaries when ruptures it leads to alveolar haemorrhage. Hemosiderin produced by lysis of RBCs is taken up by macrophage (heart failure cell) which imparts brown color to the tissue.

3. Acute hepatic congestion—Central vein and sinusoids are distended with blood. Hepatocytic degeneration is seen in central part with fatty changes in peripheral part of lobules.

4. Chronic hepatic congestion—Central part of hepatic lobules appear red brown surrounded by tan color uncongested liver (Nut Meg appearance). Centrilobular necrosis with haemorrhage and heart failure cells are also seen. Severe cases lead to central hepatic fibrosis (cardiac cirrhosis) (Fig. 9.1).

5. Chronic venous congestion of spleen (congestive splenomegaly). It is seen in right sided heart failure and portal hypertension due to cirrhosis.
   • Spleen is enlarged, congested, and cyanotic. Cut section shows gray tan surface
   • Red pulp appears congested and sinusoids are dilated with areas of haemorrhage
   • Recent and old haemorrhage when organized and haemosiderin and calcium salt is deposited, it leads to Gamna–Gandy bodies formation.

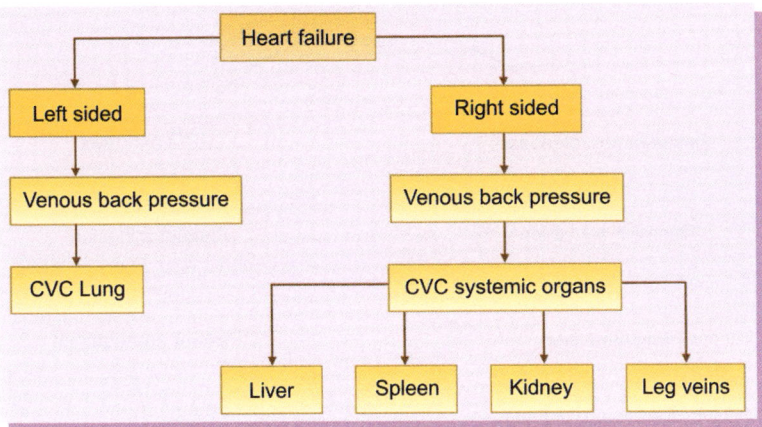

Fig. 9.11: Chronic venous congestion

6. Chronic venous congestion of kidney
   • Kidneys are enlarged, medulla appear congested
   • Tubules show degenerative changes and fatty changes. Glomeruli show mesangial proliferation

HAEMOSTASIS AND THROMBOSIS

Haemostasis is the maintenance of clot free state of blood in normal blood vessel, while inducing rapid haemostatic plug formation at the site of vascular injury (Fig. 9.12).

Thrombosis is pathologic form of haemostasis, i.e. clot formation in uninjured blood vessel or occlusive clot formation after minor trauma.

Clotting is the process of coagulation of blood *in vitro*, i.e. in test tube or outside blood vessel.

Mechanism of Haemostasis

A. Role of Endothelium in Haemostasis

1. Procoagulant Function

   • vWF synthesized by endothelium binds platelet to collagen
   • Tissue factor secreted by endothelium activate clotting factors
   • Endothelium secretes inhibitors of plasminogen activators

2. Anticoagulant Function

   • Antiplatelet effect induced by endothelial PGI (prostacyclin), nitric oxide and ADP
   • Anticoagulant effect induced by heparin like molecules and thrombomodulin

3. Fibrinolytic effect by Tissue Plasminogen Activator

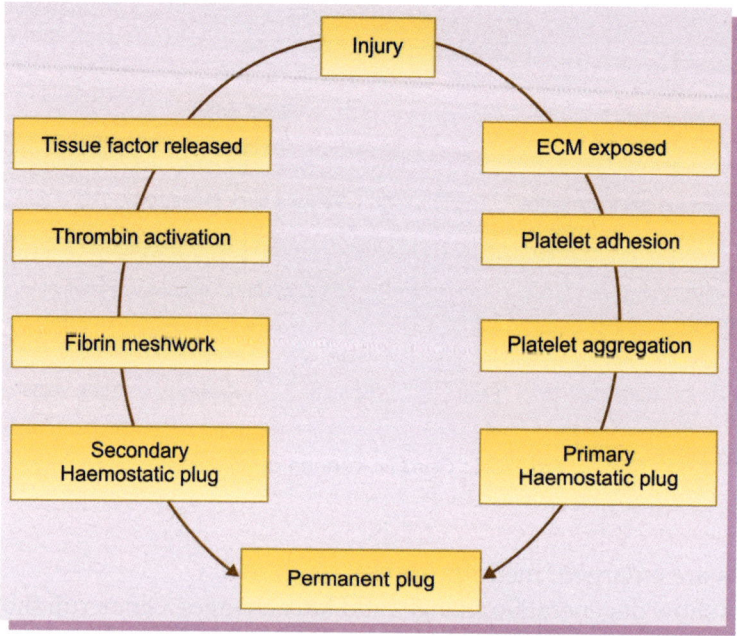

Fig. 9.12: Mechanism of haemostasis

B. *Role of Platelet in Haemostasis*

Platelet undergoes three general reactions when it comes in contact with extracellular matrix, namely

1. Platelet adhesion mediated by vWF which act as bridge between platelet receptors and exposed collagen

2. Platelet secretion is initiated by binding of agonists to platelet surface receptors and intracellular phosphorylation cascade. Dense body contains calcium which is important for coagulation pathway and ADP which is potent mediator of platelet aggregation. Platelet contains α-granules and dense bodies.

   • α-granules secretes P-selectin, adhesion molecules, fibrinogen, fibronectin, clotting factor V, VIII, platelet factor IV, PDGF, TGF-α

   • Dense bodies contain ADP, Ca^{++}, histamine, serotonin, and epinephrine

3. Platelet aggregation. ADP mediated release of thomboxane stimulates platelet aggregation leading to formation of primary haemostatic plug. Primary haemostatic plug formation is reversible unless thrombin generated by coagulation cascade converts it into secondary haemostatic plug.

C. *Role of Coagulation Cascade in Haemostasis* (Fig. 9.13)

• A series of inactivated proenzymes are activated leading to formation of thrombin, which convert insoluble fibrinogen into soluble fibrin.

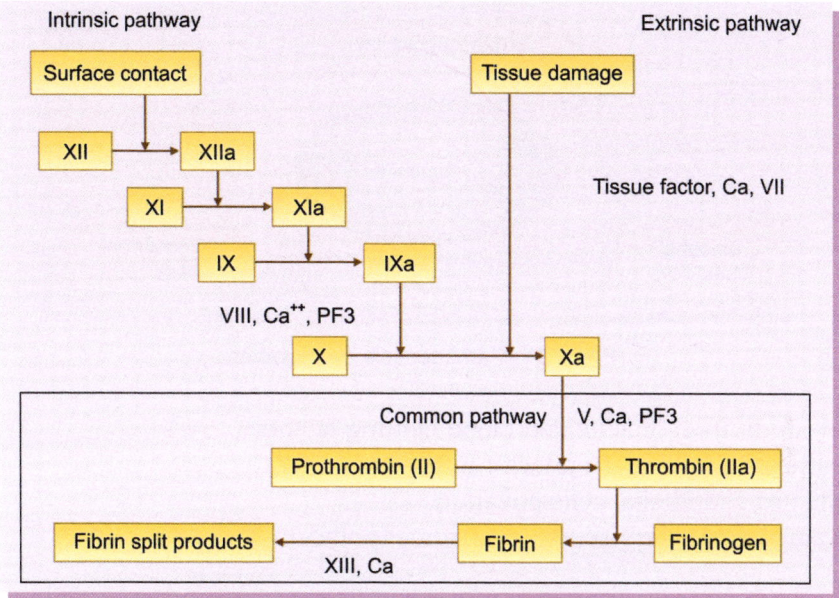

Fig. 9.13: Coagulation and fibrinolytic system

- Each reaction involves enzyme, substrate, and co factor which are assembled on phospholipid complex and held together by calcium ion, therefore clotting mechanism remains localized to the site where such assembly is present.
- Clotting is also restricted to local site by
  - Antithrombin,
  - Protein C & S, and
  - Plasmin which break down fibrin.

Pathogenesis of Thrombosis

Thrombus formation involves three factors known as Virchow's triad (Fig. 9.14)
1. Endothelial injury
2. Stasis/slowing of blood flow
3. Blood hypercoagulability

1. Endothelial Injury

Injury in heart and arteries caused by:
- Haemodynamic stress like myocardial infarction, hypertension, diabetes mellitus, atherosclerosis
- Turbulent flow of blood over scarred heart valves
- Bacterial endotoxins

2. Stasis/Slowing of Blood Flow

Stasis leads to:
- Disturbance in laminar flow of blood cells

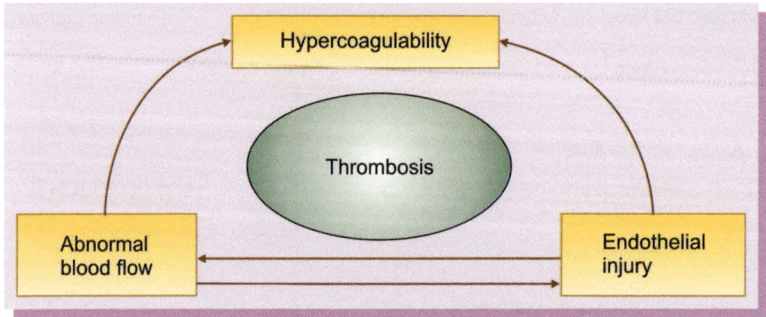

Fig. 9.14: Pathogenesis of thrombus

- Prevent dilution of activated blood clotting factors
- Retards inflow of clotting factor inhibitors
- Promotes endothelial cell activation

For example, in hyperviscocity syndrome (polycythemia vera)

3. *Hypercoagulability*

Altered coagulation pathway cause hypercoagulability states promoting thrombus formation. Causes are:

A. *Primary or Inherited*

- Mutation in factor V gene and prothrombin gene
- Deficiency of antithrombin III, protein C, protein S
- Increased homocysteine

B. *Secondary or Acquired*

- Cardiac failure
- Trauma
- Immobilization
- Cancer, DIC
- Lupus anticoagulants

Types of Thrombus

Arterial thrombus	Venous thrombus
• Develops in arteries	• Develops in veins
• Begins at the site of injury	• Develops at the site of stasis
• Grow in retrograde direction firmly attached to vessel wall	• Grow in the direction of blood flow, not firmly attached.
• Thrombus shows pale and red alternate lines of Zahn. Platelet + fibrin = pale, RBCs = red.	• Lines of Zahn are not seen, appear completely dark red.
• In heart it remains attached to the wall (mural thrombus)	

Fate of Thrombosis (Fig. 9.15)

1. Propagation: Thrombus may grow in size occupying blood vessel and its branches/tributaries.
2. Embolization: Part of the thrombus may get detached and lodged at some another distant place causing ischaemic changes.
3. Resolution: Small thrombi get dissolved by the process of thrombolysis.
4. Organization and recanalization: Fibroblast and capillaries invade the thrombus and thrombus undergoes organization. Later on organized tissue is recanalized and blood flow is restored.

Clinical Features

1. Venous Thrombosis

Develops in superficial or deep vein of lower extremities
- Cause local congestion, swelling, pain and tenderness
- Superficial thrombus rarely embolize, while deep vein thrombus from varicose vein may embolize
- Trauma, burn, injury increases procoagulant activity
- In disseminated cancers migratory thrombophlebitis develops, known as Trousseau's syndrome

2. Cardiac and Arterial Thrombosis

Dyskinetic contraction of myocardium, and endocardial and endothelial damage leads to thrombus formation.

For example in rheumatic heart disease mural thrombus develops. In atherosclerosis turbulent flow of blood favors thrombus formation.

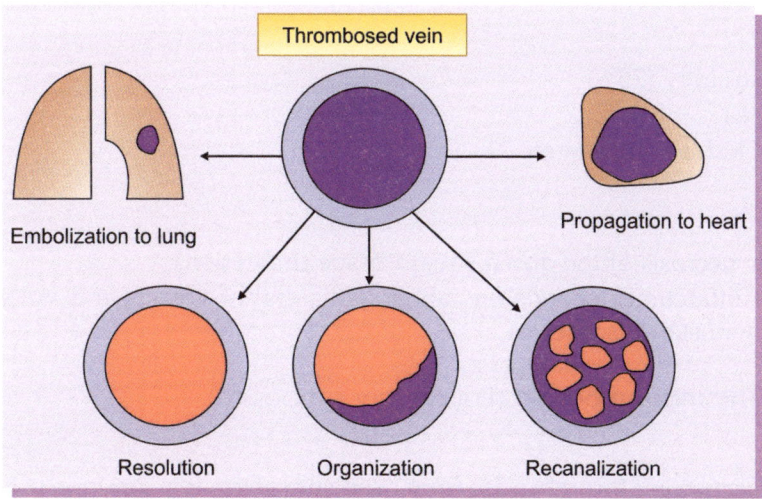

Fig. 9.15: Fate of thrombosis

EMBOLISM

Embolus is a detached intravascular solid, liquid, or gaseous mass carried by the blood to distant site from its origin. Majority (90%) of emboli are thrombus, hence solid embolism is called thromboembolism.

Classification

1. Depending on nature of matter
   - Solid
   - Liquid
   - Gaseous
2. Depending on presence of microbes
   - Bland/sterile
   - Septic
3. Depending on source
   - Cardiac
   - Arterial
   - Venous
   - Lymphatic
4. Depending on flow
   - Paradoxical (from venous to arterial circulation)
   - Retrograde (against the direction of flow)

A. Arterial Thromboembolism (Systemic embolism)

Origin of Embolus

- 80–85% arise from heart (left atrium, left ventricle, mitral valve, aortic valve)
- Rest arise from arteries (atherosclerotic plaque, aortic aneurysm)

Site of Arrest

- Lower extremity (75%)
- Brain (10%)
- Intestine, kidney, spleen, etc.

Consequences

- Ischaemic necrosis of the down stream tissue (infarction)
- Extent of infarction depends on caliber, collateral of vessels and vulnerability of tissue to withstand ischaemia

B. Venous Thromboembolism (Pulmonary embolism)

Origin of Embolus

- Ninety-five percent thrombi arise from deep vein of leg. It is common in hospitalized bedridden patients.

Site of Arrest

- In the lungs large thrombus get impacted at the bifurcation of pulmonary artery as saddle embolus
- Small multiple occlude lower lobes of the lung
- Small thrombi may pass through ventricular septal defect from right side to left side of heart and may lead to ischaemic necrosis in systemic circulation, the phenomenon known as paradoxical embolism (Fig. 9.16).

Consequences

- Most thrombi get resolved
- Sudden death due to acute corpulmonale
- Pulmonary infarction due to obstruction of arteriolar pulmonary branches
- Pulmonary haemorrhage due to obstruction of terminal pulmonary artery
- Pulmonary hypertension, chronic cor pulmonale

Fat Embolism

Obstruction of arterioles and capillaries by fat globules is known as fat embolism.

Origin

- Trauma with fracture of bones
- Nontraumatic like burn, diabetes mellitus and fatty liver.

Pathogenesis

- Mechanical theory—Physically fat globules obstruct the microvasculature
- Emulsion instability theory—Chylomicron and fatty acids break down into free fatty acids which cause endothelial injury. Endothelial injury activates platelet and

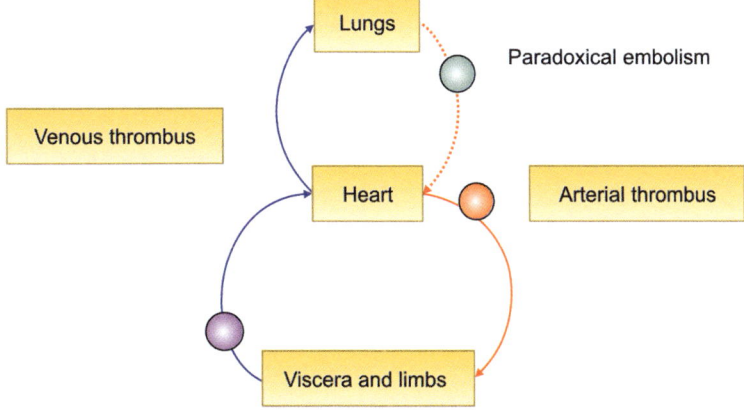

Fig. 9.16: Origin and arrest of thrombus

chemotactic factors; thereby leukocytes reach at the site. Free radicals and proteases cause vascular damage to occlude the blood vessel.

Consequences

- Pulmonary insufficiency
- Neurological symptoms, due to micro infarct and edema in brain
- Thrombocytopenia
- Death

Air Embolism

Air bubbles in the circulation can obstruct the vascular flow. This phenomenon is called air embolism. More than 100 ml of air is required to show its clinical effect.

Causes

- During obstetric procedures
- Chest wall injury
- Decompression sickness because of rapid change in pressure

Decompression Sickness

Development of air embolus due to sudden change in atmospheric pressure leads to decompression sickness.

For example, Deep sea divers when rapidly come to the surface, or passengers traveling in unpressurized aircraft at high altitude.

Pathogenesis

Under high pressure excess of nitrogen is absorbed by blood. When rapidly atmospheric pressure comes down nitrogen bubbles out and obstructs the circulation.

Consequences

- Focal ischaemia in brain and heart
- Pulmonary edema, haemorrhage and emphysema
- Chronic form of decompression sickness is known as Caisson disease. Chronic decompression sickness may lead to ischaemic necrosis of head of femur, tibia, and humerus.

Amniotic Fluid Embolism

During postpartum period (1 in 50000 deliveries) death of mother occurs, as the result of occlusion of pulmonary circulation. Amniotic fluid enters in ruptured uterine blood vessels and reaches to the heart. Cause of death is mechanical blockage of pulmonary circulation, DIC and anaphylactic reaction to amniotic fluid and haemorrhage.

Clinical Effects

- Dyspnoea, cyanosis
- Shock seizures
- Coma
- Pulmonary edema and DIC if patient survives

Pathogenesis

Amniotic fluid and its content get infused through torn placental membrane and ruptured uterine blood vessels and reach to the pulmonary microcirculation resulting in pulmonary edema, damage to alveoli and fibrin thrombi formation (disseminated intravascular coagulation).

Postmortem Finding

Squamous epithelial cells, hairs fat, mucous are found in respiratory tract and gastrointestinal tract.

Infarction

Ischaemic necrosis of tissue caused by occlusion of arterial supply or venous drainage is known as infarction.

Cause

- Ninety-nine percent of infarctions are because of thrombosis and embolism affecting arterial circulation.
- Rests are because of local vasospasm, compression of blood vessels, etc.

Organs Involved

Heart, brain, lung, GIT, spleen, etc.

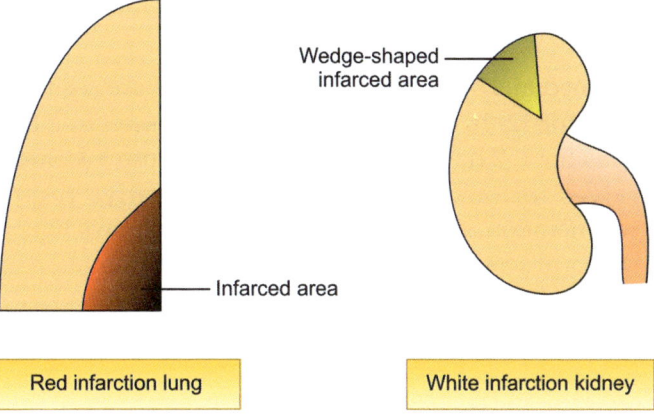

Fig. 9.17: Gross appearance of infarction

Classification

According to color of infarct

1. Red   2. White

According to presence of infection

1. Septic   2. Bland

Gross Features

- Infarced area takes wedge shape, apex being the point of obstruction, with sharp margin of hyperaemia (Fig. 9.17).
- White infarction becomes paler with time and red infarction become brown with time.

Microscopic Features

Ischaemic coagulative necrosis is seen.

Features	Red infarct	White infarct
1. Organ involved	Soft organs like lung and intestine	Solid organs like heart and kidney
2. Etiology	Due to venous obstruction	Due to arterial obstruction
3. Pathogenesis	Haemorrhage seeps into infarced area because of dual blood supply, imparting red color to the infarced tissue Previously congested tissue due to venous obstruction appears red Congested and red infarction turns brown with time, but never white	Infarced area lacks blood, because of single artery blood supply, which has been occluded, imparting white color to infarced tissue Infarced area becomes progressively pale
4. Margins	Not well-defined	Sharply defined
5. Edema	Present	Absent
6. Congestion	Present	Absent

Changes with Time

- If patient dies immediately—No microscopic changes are seen
- If patient survives for 12–18 hours—Haemorrhage is seen in infarced area
- If patient survives for 1–2 days—Inflammatory response become evident
- If patient survives for more than 1 week—Reparative response starts with parenchymal regeneration and scar formation (Brain shows liquefactive necrosis)
- Septic infarct shows abscess formation and greater inflammation which later on get organized

Factors Affecting Infarction

1. Nature of vascular supply. If alternate blood supply is present, for example in lung liver, forearm and hand, then no infarction is seen.

2. If rate of development of occlusion is slow then no infarction is seen.

3. Vulnerability of tissue to withstand hypoxia.
   - Neurons show irreversible changes if ischaemia persist for 3–4 minutes
   - Myocardial cells dies within 20 to 30 seconds after ischaemia
   - Fibroblasts remain viable for hours of ischaemia

4. Oxygen content of blood. Patient suffering from congestive heart failure and anaemia are more vulnerable to suffer from ischaemic necrosis.

10

Hypertension and Shock

HYPERTENSION

A patient is said to be hypertensive when his systolic blood pressure is more than 140 mmHg and diastolic blood pressure is more than 90 mmHg.

Normal Blood Pressure

- Systolic 100–140 mmHg
- Diastolic 60–90 mmHg

Hypertension is a Risk Factor

- Coronary heart disease
- Cerebrovascular accidents
- Heart failure
- Renal failure

Classification

1. Essential or Primary Hypertension

In 90–95% cases when the cause of hypertension is not identifiable, then it is labeled as primary hypertension. Factors which are related to its development are:

- *Genetic factors:* Familial clustering is seen and high prevalence is seen in twins.
- *Racial factors:* Black persons are more affected than white.
- *Environmental factors:* Environmental factors like salt intake, obesity, stressful conditions have been found to be associated with hypertension.
- *Food and habit:* Cigarettes smoking, high fatty diet, alcohol, sedentary lifestyle increases the risk of development of hypertension.

2. Secondary Hypertension

In 5–10% cases hypertension is secondary to some other disease. Like

A. *Renal Disease*

- Acute glomerulonephritis
- Chronic renal failure
- Polycystic disease of kidney
- Renal artery stenosis
- Renin producing tumours

B. *Endocrine Disorders*

- Adrenocortical dysfunction
- Exogenous hormones
- Pheochromocytoma
- Acromegaly
- Hypo/hyperthyroidism

C. *Cardiovascular Disease*

- Coarctation of aorta
- Polyarteritis nodosa (PAN)
- Increased cardiac output
- Increased intravascular volume

D. *Neurogenic Disorders*

- Psychogenic
- Increased intracranial pressure
- Acute stress

Regulation of Normal Blood Pressure (Fig. 10.1)

Role of Heart

Blood pressure is a product of cardiac output and peripheral resistance. Cardiac output depends on heart rate, contractility and blood volume. Heart rate and contractility are cardiac factors while blood volume is regulated by sodium homeostasis.

Role of Kidney

- *Sodium homeostasis:* It is maintained by release of aldosterone through renin angiotensin mechanism and tubular reabsorption at proximal tubules.
- *Renin angiotensin system:* Activated by renal ischaemia, angiotensin is produced; it stimulates adrenals to secrete aldosterone and catecholamine, thereby constricting arterioles, so that peripheral resistance is increased.

Role of Vasodepressor Material

A number of vasodepressor substances like prostaglandins and nitric oxide counter balance the effect of vasopressors.

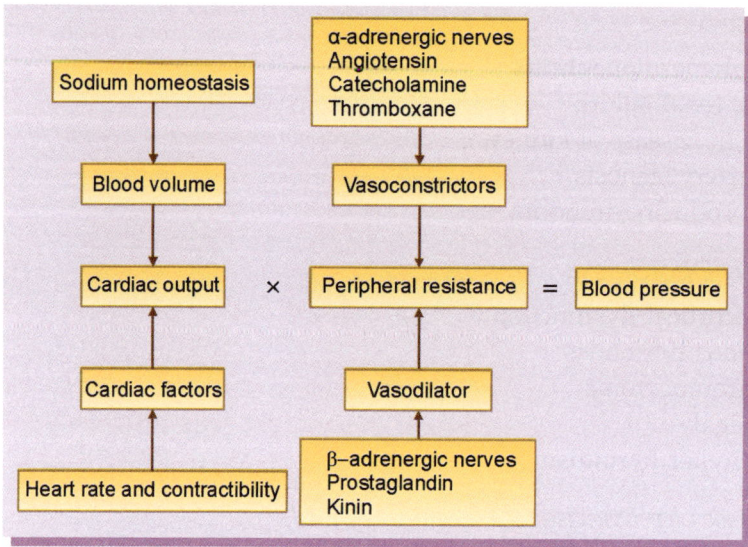

Fig. 10.1: Regulation of normal blood pressure

Natriureteric Factors

Natriureteric peptides are secreted by atrial and ventricular myocardium, which cause sodium excretion and vasodilatation.

Neural Factors

α-adrenergic nerves are vasoconstrictors while β-adrenergic are vasodilators.

Pathogenesis of Hypertension

Two overlapping pathways have been proposed to understand the mechanism involved in the development of hypertension.

I. Renal Retention of Excess Sodium

Defect in renal sodium homeostasis is primary cause of hypertension. Decreased sodium excretion results in salt and water retention leading to increased blood volume and increased cardiac output. Increased cardiac output results in hypertension.

II. Vasoconstriction and Vascular Hypertrophy

Increased peripheral resistance due to

A. Functional Vasoconstriction by

- Behavioral/neurogenic factors
- Increased release of vasoactive amines
- Increased sensitivity of smooth muscle cells

B. *Structural Changes in Vessel Wall Brought about by*

Vasoconstrictors, acting as growth factors for smooth muscle hypertrophy, hyperplasia and matrix deposition in chronic vasoconstriction.

Conclusion: It is a complex disorder and a multifactorial disease.

Morphological Changes

Hypertension affects mainly blood vessels, heart, kidneys and central nervous system.

1. Blood Vessels

Following changes are seen in blood vessels
- Hyaline arteriosclerosis
- Hyperplastic arteriosclerosis
- Necrotizing arteriolitis

A. Hyaline Arteriosclerosis

It is physiological but it is accelerated in hypertension. There is leakage of components of plasma, immunoglobulin, compliment, fibrin and lipids in intima. Morphological features are
- Narrowed lumen with thickened vascular wall
- Homogenous pink hyaline material in the intima and media

B. Hyperplastic Arteriosclerosis

In malignant hypertension and toxemia of pregnancy endothelial damage leads to increased permeability. Intimal thickening may show three types of changes
   i. *Onion skin changes*: Concentric laminated thickening due to smooth muscle hyperplasia give rise to this type of characteristic appearance.
   ii. *Mucinous intimal thickening:* There is deposition of amorphous material in intima.
   iii. *Fibrous intimal thickening:* Collagen bundle, elastic fibre and hyaline material is seen in intimal layer.

C. Necrotizing Arteriolitis

In malignant hypertension when there is sudden rise in blood pressure, direct damage to vessel occurs. Blood vessel shows fibrinoid necrosis and neutrophilic exudate in adventitia.

2. Heart

Hypertension of prolonged duration potentiates ischaemic heart disease, cerebro vascular strokes and renal failure. There is hypertrophy of heart, chiefly left ventricle.

3. *Kidney*

A. *Benign Nephrosclerosis*

Benign hypertension leads to benign nephrosclerosis. Long-standing cases show mild proteinuria and hyaline casts.

Gross features
Renal cortex is shrunken with adherent capsule over it, giving granular grain leather appearance.

Microscopic features
- Small arteries and arterioles show hyaline arteriosclerosis and intimal thickening
- Parenchyma shows shrinkage of glomeruli with periglomerular fibrosis and finally total sclerosis. Tubules show atrophy and interstitium shows fibrosis.

B. *Malignant Nephrosclerosis*

It is seen in malignant hypertension. It may occur superimposed over benign nephrosclerosis or alone. Renal function is deranged with haematuria and proteinuria.

Gross features
- In pure form of malignant nephrosclerosis kidneys are enlarged with pin point petechial haemorrhage giving rise to flea bitten appearance.
- When superimposed over benign nephrosclerosis, kidneys are shrunken.

Microscopic features
- Blood vessels show features of necrotizing arteriolitis and hyperplastic arteriosclerosis.
- Parenchyma shows tubular atrophy with fine interstitial fibrosis and focal areas of infarction.

4. *Central Nervous System*

Cerebrovascular infarction, haemorrhage, ischaemic attacks and subarachnoid haemorrhage are seen.

SHOCK

Definition

It is a clinical state of cardiovascular collapse, characterized by systemic hypoperfusion and cellular hypoxia.

Causes

- Severe haemorrhage
- Extensive burn
- Large myocardial infarction

- Massive pulmonary embolism
- Microbial sepsis

Classification (Based on etiology)

1. Cardiogenic

- Myocardial infarction
- Ventricular rupture
- Pulmonary embolism

2. Hypovolemic

- Haemorrhage due to trauma/surgery
- Fluid loss due to vomiting, diarrhea, burn

3. Systemic Microbial Infection (Septic)

- Gram-negative bacterial endotoxins (common)
- Gram-positive exotoxins (less common)

4. Neurogenic

- Spinal cord injury (loss of vascular tone)

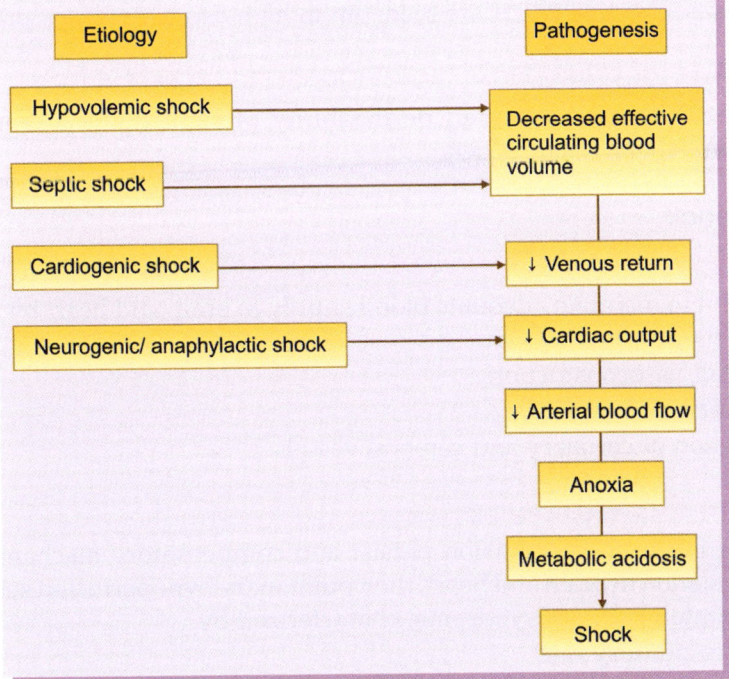

Fig. 10.2: Etiopathogenesis of shock

5. Anaphylactic

IgE mediated hypersensitivity reactions

Pathogenesis (Fig. 10.2)

1. Pathogenesis of Cardiogenic Shock

Acute circulatory failure with sudden fall in cardiac output results in decreased effective circulating blood volume. Reduced oxygen supply which induces tissue hypoxia and metabolic acidosis leads to shock.

2. Pathogenesis of Hypovolemic Shock

Decreased plasma volume occur due to loss of fluid in vomiting, diarrhoea, burn and injury. Tissue hypoxia leads to metabolic acidosis resulting into membrane damage and cell death. Failure of precapillary sphincter results in peripheral pooling of blood which further aggravates the condition.

3. Pathogenesis of Septic Shock

Cell wall of gram-negative bacilli is composed of lipopolysaccharide (LPS), which binds to LPS binding protein forming an LPS-BP complex. This complex binds to CD-14 receptors present on inflammatory cells and release cytokines. Cytokines cause endothelial injury. In low doses cytokines produce acute inflammation, while in moderate doses systemic effects are seen, but in high doses cytokines produce shock.

4. Pathogenesis of Neurogenic and Anaphylactic Shock

Peripheral pooling and increased permeability of capillaries, is responsible for neurogenic and anaphylactic shock.

Stages of Shock

A. Nonprogressive Shock (Reversible)

It is an attempt to maintain adequate blood supply to brain and heart by activation of reflex compensatory mechanism, i.e.
- Wide spread vasoconstriction
- Fluid conservation by kidney
- Vasodilatation of coronary and cerebral vessels

B. Progressive, Decompensated Shock

If underlying cause of hypotension persist and compensatory mechanisms fails to maintain circulation in brain and heart, then pulmonary hypoperfusion sets in, leading to acute respiratory distress syndrome, characterized by
- Increased respiratory rate
- Cellular hypoxia activates anaerobic glycolysis leading to metabolic acidosis
- Anoxia to liver also causes acidosis

C. Decompensated Shock (Irreversible)

Anoxic damage to lung, kidney, brain, heart leads to
- Progressive fall in blood pressure
- Respiratory distress syndrome
- Severe metabolic acidosis
- Ischaemic death of brain, heart and kidney

Morphological Features

Hypoxia results in degeneration and necrosis of major organs like brain, heart lung and kidney.
- Brain shows neuronal degeneration and gliosis
- Heart shows ischaemic necrosis
- Lung shows congestion, edema, fibrosis, thrombus formation
- Kidney shows acute tubular necrosis
- Adrenal shows haemorrhage
- GIT shows haemorrhagic necrosis and secondary infections
- Liver shows fatty changes and central necrosis

Clinical Features

- Hypotension
- Decreased body temperature
- Tachycardia
- Shallow and decreased respiratory rate
- Pale face, sunken eyes, cold and clammy skin, weakness
- Oliguria and later on diuresis
- Stupor turns into coma and finally death supervenes

11

Nutritional Diseases

DEFINITION

Many natural constituents in food threat the human health like coffee, nutmeg, basil which contains many caner causing natural compounds. At the same time, additives like pesticides, food preservatives, color, and sweeteners also affect our health. Contamination of food with microorganisms, toxins and metal are responsible for various health hazards. However, much significant health problem associated with nutrition is deficiency diseases due to malnourishment.

Causes of Nutritional Deficiency Diseases in General

A. *Primary Deficiency*

It is due to lack or decreased amount of essential nutrient in food.

B. *Secondary Deficiency*

It is due to other factors which interfere with
1. Ingestion of food
   - For example, GIT diseases, anorexia, alcoholism, food allergy, vomiting
2. Absorption of nutrients
   - For example, increased motility, achlorhydria, biliary disease
3. Utilization of nutrients
   - For example, liver dysfunction, malignancy, hypothyroidism
4. Increased excretion nutrients
   - For example, polyuria, lactation
5. Increased demand for nutrition
   - For example, pregnancy, hyperthyroidism

Pathogenesis of Nutritional Deficiency Diseases

Persistent deficiency of nutrients depletes the body stores. Biochemical alterations due to deficiency of nutrients lead to the morphological and functional changes. Such changes can be reversed back if adequate nutrients are made available (Fig. 11.1).

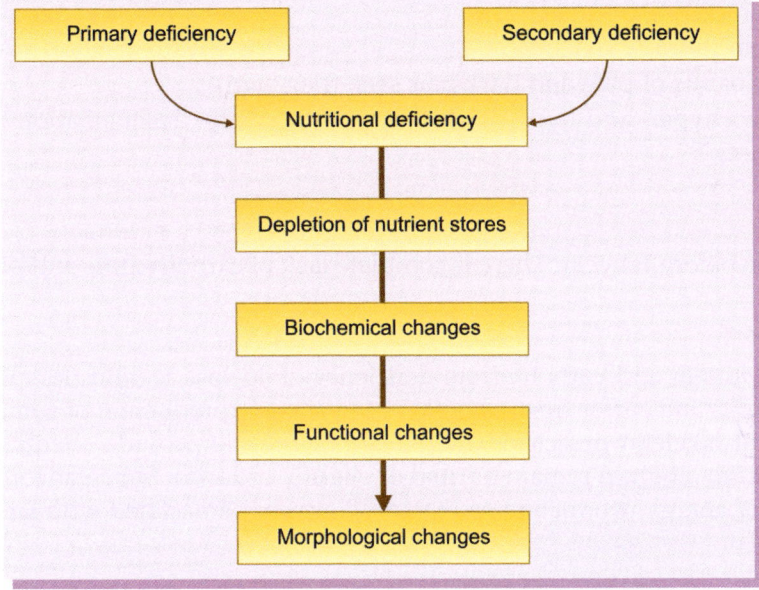

Fig. 11.1: Pathogenesis of nutritional deficiency disease

PROTEIN ENERGY MALNUTRITION (PEM)

Definition

Inadequate consumption of protein and/or carbohydrate results in a range of clinical symptoms, like kwashiorkor and marasmus.

Kwashiorkor

It is common between the age group of 3 months to 3 years. It develops when child consumes diet deficient in protein but with sufficient calories. For example, during weaning period when child consumes only piece of bread but no protein (pulses or vegetable) at all. Such children are susceptible for various infections like respiratory or intestinal infections, which further aggravate the condition.

Pathogenesis

Severe protein deficiency leads to hypoalbuminaemia resulting in generalized edema. Because of edema, weight of the child may be almost normal but growth of body is affected. Visceral protein compartment (liver) is more affected than somatic protein compartment (skeletal muscle) producing hypoalbuminaemia.

Clinical Features

- Growth failure with peripheral edema
- Muscle wasting but preserved adipose tissue

- Fatty liver with hepatomegaly
- Low serum protein, anaemia
- Alternate bands of pale and dark hair seen (flag sign)
- Skin shows hyper- and hypopigmentation with patchy desquamation (flaky paint appearance)

Marasmus

It is common before 1st year. There is complete lack of carbohydrate and protein both.

Pathogenesis

Because of protein and carbohydrate deficiency child lose weight (less than 60% of normal weight) and suffer from growth retardation and reduction of somatic protein compartment (skeletal muscles). Catabolism of muscle provide adequate proteins therefore serum albumin remain normal or slightly reduced. Subcutaneous fat is also mobilized for energy production so that child appears emaciated with large head.

Clinical Features

- Growth failure with emaciated extremities and large head (monkey like face)
- Wasting of muscles as well as adipose tissue
- No fatty changes in liver
- Low serum protein, anaemia
- Flag sign is not observed

VITAMINS

Definition

Vitamins are organic substances which cannot be synthesized by body and are essential for maintenance of normal structure and functions of cells.

Fat Soluble Vitamins

1. Vitamin A
2. Vitamin D
3. Vitamin E
4. Vitamin K

These are absorbed from intestine in the presence of bile salt and intact pancreatic function. Deficiency usually occurs due to secondary causes.

Water Soluble Vitamins

1. Vitamin C
2. Vitamin B complex
   - Vitamin B_1 (thiamine)

- Vitamin B_2 (niacin)
- Vitamin B_6 (pyridoxine)
- Vitamin B_{12} (cynocobalamine)

Vitamin A

Vitamin A includes group of related compounds like retinal, retinol, and retinoid acid.

Sources

- Retinol is present in animal derived food like egg, butter, milk, liver, and kidney.
- Carotinoids are beta carotene found in yellow and green leafy vegetables and fruits. These are converted into retinol by body.

Functions

A. Vision

Retinol is stored as retinyl in body and broken into retinol whenever needed. Retinol 11 [*cis*] form is used for rhodopsin production, a dim light vision pigment. Inadequate availability of retinol results in impaired dark adaptation, condition known as night blindness.

B. Epithelium

Retinoic acid is required for orderly differentiation of mucus secreting glands. Deficiency leads to:

- Xerophthalmia (dry eye), Xerosis (dry conjunctiva) Bitot's spot (collection of keratin debris), keratomalacia.

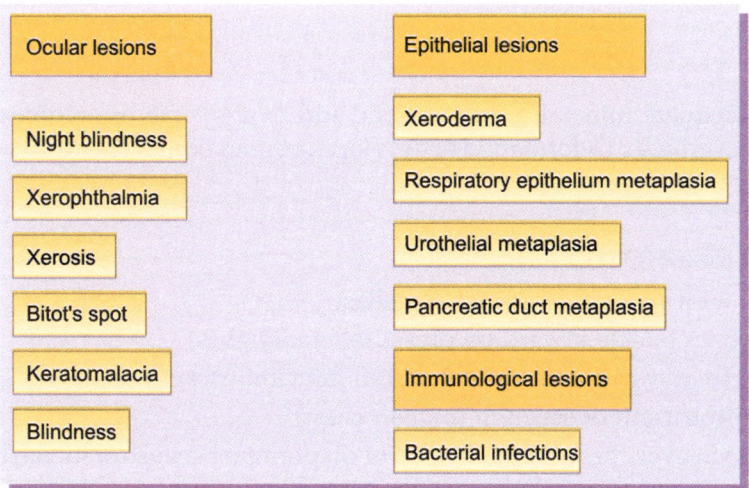

Fig. 11.2: Vitamin A deficiency lesions

- Squamous metaplasia of upper respiratory tract epithelium, follicular dyskeratosis, xeroderma.

C. Immunity

It also stimulates immune system. Therefore deficiency predisposes to bacterial infections.

Vitamin D

Vitamin D exits in two forms
1. Vitamin D_2 (calciferol). This is synthesized from plants and yeast precursors.
2. Vitamin D_3 (cholecalciferol). It is formed in skin by sunlight.

Sources

Food source is fortified cereals, fish liver oil, egg, butter milk.
Vitamin D_2 and vitamin D_3 are converted into active form calcitriol by liver and kidney.

Function

Vitamin D is necessary for formation, growth and repair of bones. It also enhances immune function and improves muscle strength.

Deficiency Diseases

- Rickets in children
- Osteomalacia in adults
- Tetany

Bone Changes

There is inadequate mineralization of bone and overgrowth of epiphyseal cartilage affecting bone growth. Deformation of developing bones occurs due to loss of structural rigidity.

In Children (Rickets) (Fig. 11.3)

- Soft skull with space between frontenelles
- Parietal bones buckle inward by pressure (craniotabes)
- Overgrowth of cartilage at costochondral junction (ricketic rosary)
- Anterior protrusion of sternum (pigeon chest)
- Grove is seen over chest at the margins of diaphragm because of inward pull during respiration (Harrison's sulcus)
- Bowleg and knock knee because of sustained body weight over both knees

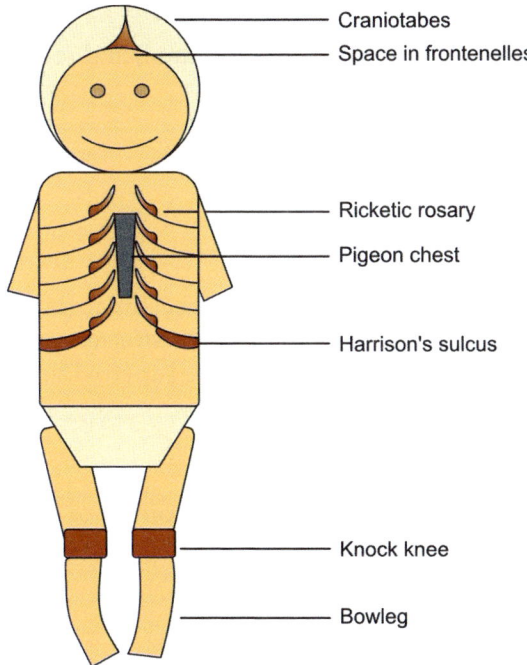

Craniotabes
Space in frontenelles
Ricketic rosary
Pigeon chest
Harrison's sulcus
Knock knee
Bowleg

Fig. 11.3: Lesions in rickets

In Adult (Osteomalacia)

In adult since bone growth has been completed, therefore features are related with derangement of bone remodeling which occurs throughout the life. Poorly mineralized osteoid tissue is not able to withstand body weight resulting in deformation and become vulnerable to get fractured. Features of osteomalacia are:

• Increased convexity of lumbar vertebrae (lumber lordosis)
• Muscular weakness
• Pathological fracture

Causes of deficiency
• Inadequate exposure to sunlight
• Breastfed infants
• Malabsorption states
• Kidney and liver disorders
• Anticonvulsant drugs and rifampicin

Biochemical changes
• Decreased active metabolites of vitamin D
• Serum calcium is normal or decreased
• Serum phosphorus is decreased
• Serum alkaline phosphatase activity is increased

Vitamin E

It is fat soluble compound (4-tocoferol and 4-tocoretinol) and requires intact pancreatic and biliary function for its absorption.

Sources

Vegetables, grains, nuts, oils, fish and meat

Function

It acts as antioxidant and prevents cellular and subcellular damage due to oxidants and free radicals. Neurons with long axon are more affected producing neurological manifestations. Red cells are also vulnerable because superoxide radicals are generated during oxygenation of haemoglobin.

Pathological changes due to deficiency

- Degeneration of neurons in posterior column of spinal cord
- Demyelination of axons of peripheral nerves
- Demineralization of skeletal muscles
- Degeneration of retinal pigment
- Decreased lifespan of RBCs

Clinical Features

- Depressed tendon reflexes
- Ataxia, dysarthria
- Loss of positional and vibration sense
- Muscle weakness and impairment of vision

Vitamin K

Sources

1. Vitamin K_1
   - Derived from green leafy vegetables
2. Vitamin K_2
   - Produced endogenously by bacterial flora of intestine, therefore very small quantity is required

Functions

Vitamin K is a cofactor for liver microsomal carboxylase, which causes
- Carboxylation of glutamyl residue of protein to carboxyglutamylate (Factor II, VII, IX, X). Carboxylation provide calcium binding site for calcium dependent interaction of clotting factors
- Carboxylation of osteocalcin increases calcium and osteocalcin interaction and favors bone calcification
- Vitamin K dependent carboxylation activates Protein C and S

Causes of deficiency
- In neonatal period when intestinal flora are not well developed, liver reserves are low and breast milk is poor source of vitamin K
- Biliary obstruction, diffuse liver disease
- Malabsorption syndrome
- Antibiotic therapy
- Anticoagulant therapy

Clinical manifestations
Bleeding diathesis due to hypoprothrombinaemia
- Haematoma
- Haematuria
- Melena
- Bleeding gums
- Ecchymoses

Vitamin C

Sources

Vitamin C is abundant in citrus fruits and fresh vegetables. Vitamin C is water soluble and destroyed on boiling.

Functions

1. Role in Collagen Synthesis

- It accelerates hydroxylation and amidation reaction in synthesis of ground substances like osteoid, chondroitin sulphate, dentine and cement of vascular endothelium.
- It activates prolyl and lysyl hydroxylases for hydroxylation of procollagen

2. Role as Anti-oxidant

- Neutralize effect of free radicals, stabilizes folic acid
- Regenerate anti-oxidant form of vitamin E and reduces oxidation of LDL cholesterol in atherosclerosis, there by preventing its progress
- Role in iron absorption and its storage

Deficiency Disease Scurvy is Characterized by

1. Haemorrhage

- Purpura and ecchymoses in skin and mucus membrane
- Gingival swelling and periodontal infections
- Subperiosteal haemorrhage and bleeding in joints
- Rarely retrobulbar, subarachnoid and intracerebral haemorrhage

2. Skeletal Changes

- Weak scorbutic bone
- Bowleg
- Depressed sternum and scorbutic rosary

3. Delayed Wound Healing

Due to deficient collagen synthesis

4. Anaemia

Due to haemorrhage, folic acid deficiency and iron deficiency

Vitamin B Complex

Vitamin B was initially coined for beriberi (vital mineral B), now used for group of essential compounds biochemically different but occurs together in food like leafy vegetables, cereals, yeast, liver, milk, etc.

Vitamin B_1 (Thiamine)

Sources

Raw food, destroyed by tea, coffee and lost by washing

Functions

- It acts as coenzyme for oxidative decarboxylation of α-keto acids leading to synthesis of ATP
- Act as a cofactor for transketolase in pentose phosphate pathway for synthesis of fat from carbohydrate
- It maintains the integrity and function of nerves

Deficiency Diseases

Due to incomplete combustion of carbohydrate leading to decreased ATP production and accumulation of pyruvic acid

1. Dry beriberi (peripheral neuritis) characterized by weakness, pareasthesia and sensory loss.
2. Wet beriberi (cardiac) characterized by generalized edema, serous effusion and congestion of viscera.
3. Cerebral beriberi (Wernicke-Korsakoff's syndrome) characterized by degeneration, demyelination and haemorrhage in brain.

Vitamin B_2 (Riboflavin)

Sources

Plant and animal food. It is yellow-orange in color hence used for food coloring

Function

Act as cytochrome oxidase enzyme in cellular respiration.

Deficiency Manifestations

- Ocular—Vascularization of cornea leads to photophobia
- Oral—Angular cheilitis, stomatitis, glossitis
- Skin—Seborrheic dermatitis of nasolabial fold, scrotum, vulva

Vitamin B_3 (Nicotinic acid or niacin)

Sources

All animal and plant food contain niacin in abundance. In maize niacin is present in bound form, hence not absorbable.

Function

Biologically active derivative nicotinamide is essential component of NAD (Nicotinamide adenine dinucleotide) and NADP (Nicotinamide adenine dinucleotide phosphate)

Deficiency Disease is Pellagra (Means Rough Skin): It is Characterized by

- Dermatitis: Sun exposed skin develops erythema, chronic dermatitis with blisters.
- Diarrhea: Lesions similar to skin develop in mucous membrane of GIT causing vomiting to diarrhea.
- Dementia: Degeneration of brain and spinal tract leads to dementia, peripheral neuritis, visual and auditory disturbances.

Vitamin B_6 (Pyridoxine)

Sources

It is widely distributed in all animal and plant food in three forms:
Pyridoxine, pyridoxal and pyridoxamine

Functions

- Metabolic function—Fat, protein and amino acid metabolism
- Transmission of neural impulses
- In immune function

Deficiency Manifestations

- Dermatitis
- Angular cheilitis and stomatitis
- Glossitis
- Sideroblastic anaemia
- Convulsion in infant

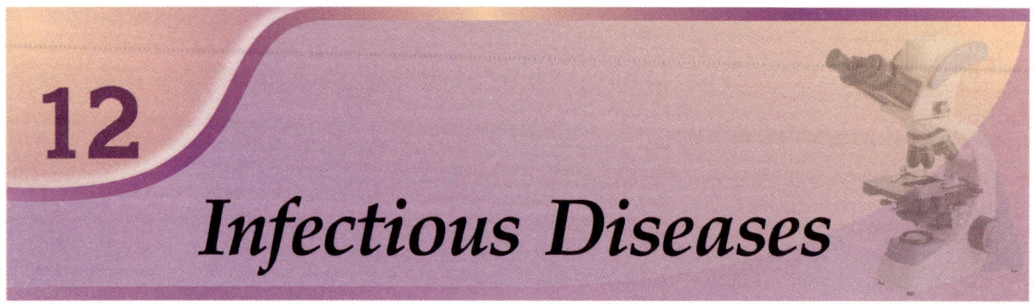

Infectious Diseases

TUBERCULOSIS

Tuberculosis is specific type of chronic granulomatous inflammation. It is delayed type IV hypersensitivity reaction to poorly digestible organism resulting into characteristic granuloma formation.

Causative Organism

Mycobacterium tuberculosis, occasionally atypical mycobacterium.

Incidence

It is common in poor countries of Africa, Latin America and Asia.

Mode of Transmission

Bacteria enter into human body through
- Inhalation
- Ingestion
- Inoculation
- Transplacental route

Spread in Body

- Local spread in surrounding tissue
- Lymphatic spread to lymph nodes
- Haematogenous spread to different organs
- Through natural passages like respiratory tract, gastrointestinal tract and urinary tract to adjoining areas

Pathogenesis

It is host response to the organism in the form of cell mediated hypersensitivity reaction type IV. Depending on type of tissue response, it consists of two types.

1. *Primary Tuberculosis*

The person who has not been exposed previously or immunized, when infected by M. tubercular bacilli first time, shows primary immune response and develop primary tuberculosis/Ghon's complex (Fig. 12.1).

Ghon's Complex (Primary Tuberculosis) is a Triad Consisting of

- Lesion produced at the site of entry
- Regional lymph nodes involvement and
- Inflammation of draining lymphatics

Most common tissues involved in primary complex are lungs, hilar lymph node and the draining lymphatics. Lesion in the lung is a sub pleural pneumonitis in lower lobe. Draining lymphatics contain macrophages with bacilli. Hilar and tracheobronchial lymph node shows caseative necrosis. Other tissues involved may be cervical lymph nodes, tonsils, intestine and mesenteric lymph nodes.

Fate of Primary Tuberculosis

1. Healing—Lesion may heal with fibrosis and later on get calcified
2. Progressive—Caseous material may be drained through bronchi to other parts of lung
3. Miliary—Bacilli may enter into the circulation and may produce diffuse minute lesion in other organ like liver, spleen, kidney and brain.
4. Reactivation—Dormant bacilli get activated under certain circumstances such as low immunity or increased hypersensitivity.

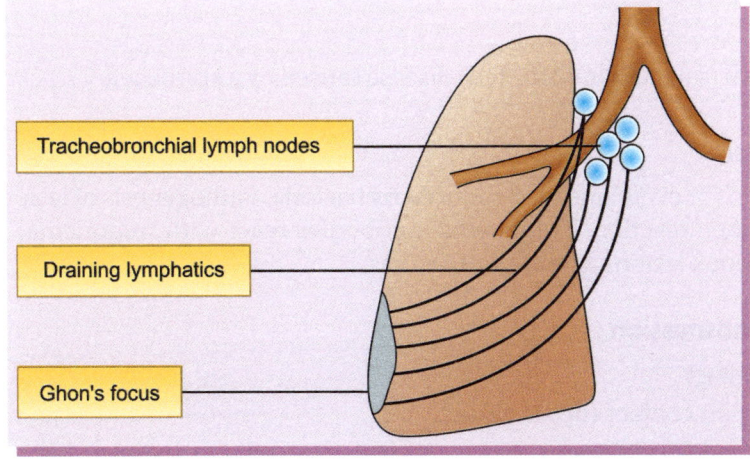

Fig. 12.1: Ghon's complex

2. Secondary Tuberculosis

Apical area of lung where oxygen tension is high favors the development of secondary tuberculosis. The lesion reach through haematogenous spread and form typical chronic granulomatous lesion with caseation.

Fate of Secondary Tuberculosis

- Lesion heals with scar formation and calcification
- Lesion may coalesce to produce fibrocaseous tuberculosis, cavitations, tubercular pneumonia, or miliary tuberculosis

Complications

- Extension of lesion to the pleura leads to pleural effusion
- Aneurysm of artery crossing cavity get ruptured and produces haemoptysis
- Deposition of caseous material over pleura produce empyema
- Thickening of pleura occur with adhesion formation

Clinical Features

Respiratory symptoms
- Productive cough
- Haemoptysis
- Pleural effusion
- Dyspnoea

Systemic symptoms
Fever, night sweats, fatigue, loss of weight, and appetite

SYPHILIS

Etiology

It is a venereal (sexually transmitted) disease caused by a spirochete *Treponema pallidum*.

Pathogenesis

No endotoxins or exotoxins are produced by bacteria. Pathogenesis of lesions is because of host immune reaction. Treponemal antibodies react with treponemal antigen and produce various lesions at different lesions.

Mode of Transmission

1. Sexual contact
2. Intimate skin contact (lip, tongue)
3. Infected blood transfusion
4. To fetus through transplacental route

Clinical Stages

1. *Primary Syphilis*

Painless papules develop at genitals/extra genital region accompanied by lymphadenopathy, which heals after 2–4 weeks of exposure.

2. *Secondary Syphilis (Infective stage)*

- Mucocutaneous lesions are seen in oral cavity, palm, hands and feet
- Macular and pustular patches over skin of penis/vulva are most infectious
- Papular lesions over penis and vulva later on develop elevated plaques called condyloma lata along with lymphadenopathy. These lesions develop 2–3 months after exposure.

3. *Tertiary Syphilis*

Syphilitic gumma, diffuse cardiac and neurological lesions are seen 2–3 years after exposure. At this stage patient is less infective.

Syphilitic Gumma

It is localized, solitary, rubbery lesion with central necrosis in liver, testis, bones and brain. Microscopically coagulative necrosis with macrophages, lymphocytes, plasma cells, giant cells and fibroblasts are seen.

Diffuse Cardiac Lesions

Thoracic aorta may show aneurysm, aortic regurgitation and narrowing of coronary ostea.

Diffuse Neurological Lesions

Meningovascular syphilis, tabes dorsalis and general paresis may be seen.

Congenital Syphilis

It occurs through transplacental transmission of infective organism to the fetus of more than 16 weeks old. Before 16th week Treponema do not invade placental tissue or fetus.

Clinical Features

Premature death, late abortion or stillbirth of fetus may occur. If fetus survive then lesion persist as latent infection and become apparent at infant or later age.

At infant age
- Mucocutaneous lesion develops
- Bone lesions (osteochondritis and periostitis)
- Collapse of bridge of nose creates saddle nose deformity
- Liver and lung shows diffuse interstitial fibrosis

At later age
- Interstitial keratitis and choroiditis
- Hutchinson's teeth (small widely spaces peg-shaped incisors)
- Eighth nerve deafness (tertiary syphilis)

Laboratory Investigations

1. Demonstration of *T. pallidum* by
   - Dark field microscopy
   - Fluorescent antibody technique
   - Silver impregnation technique
2. Detection of treponemal antibodies by
   - Reiter protein complement fixation test (RPCF)
   - *Treponema pallidum* immobilization test (TPI)
   - Fluorescent treponemal antibodies (FTA)
   - Treponemal passive haem agglutination test (TPHA)
3. Detection of Wassermann antibodies by
   - Wassermann compliment fixation test (CFT)
   - Venereal disease research laboratory test (VDRL)
   - Rapid plasma reagin (RPR)

TYPHOID (ENTERIC FEVER)

Enteric fever is food and waterborn disease of developing countries where sanitation and water hygiene is poor.

Etiology

It is an acute infection caused by *Salmonella typhi/paratyphi* (Gram-negative bacilli) *Salmonella* possess somatic antigen "O" and flagellar antigen "H"

Pathogenesis (Fig. 12.2)

- Ingestion of food or water contaminated with feces of infected person leads to entry of bacilli in intestine
- Bacteria colonize in lymphoid Peyer's patches of intestine resulting in hyperplasia of lymphoid tissue
- Eventually Peyer's patches ulcerate resulting in spread of bacteria throughout the body by lymphatics and blood
- In the gall bladder bacteria grow in bile juice and reenters in intestine through bile

Clinical Features

- Typhoid shows characteristic fever pattern (sustained and gradually rising fever) with profuse sweating and malaise.

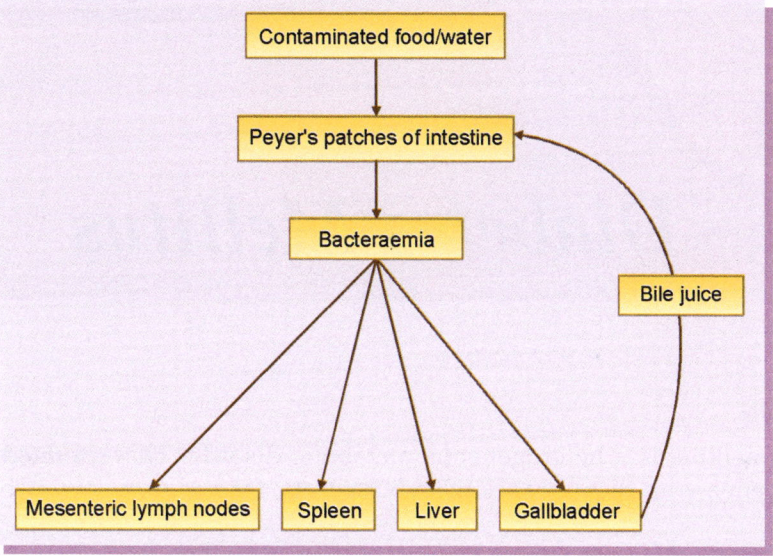

Fig. 12.2: Pathogenesis of enteric fever

- Rose color rashes and spots over skin
- Diarrhea, hepatomegaly, and pain abdomen
- Relative bradycardia, epistaxis, headache, etc.

Clinical Course of Disease

- 1st week (Bacteraemia): Fever, chills, headache, pain abdomen
- 2nd week (Lymphoid hyperplasia): Rashes, diarrhea, hepatosplenomegaly
- 3rd week (Ulceration): Intestinal bleeding, shock, melena
- 4th week (Bacteria in bile): Resolution, relapse with cholecystitis

Complications

- Bleeding and melena, perforation with septicemia
- Metastatic abscess, osteomyelitis, nephritis, meningitis
- Chronic cholecystitis

Laboratory Investigations

- Complete blood count shows leucopenia, relative lymphocytosis
- Blood culture in 1st week for isolation of salmonella.
- Widal test, typhoid ELISA test for detection of IgG and IgM antibodies

13
Diabetes Mellitus

DEFINITION

Diabetes mellitus is a heterogeneous metabolic disorder characterized by chronic hyperglycemia with disturbances of carbohydrate, fat and protein metabolism.

Classification

1. **Type I diabetes mellitus** (Insulin dependent DM or juvenile onset diabetes)
   i. Type IA DM (Immune mediated) β cell destruction and absolute insulin deficiency.
   ii. Type IB DM (Idiopathic)
2. **Type II DM** (Noninsulin dependent DM or maturity onset diabetes) insulin resistance with relative insulin deficiency.
3. **Other** specific types of diabetes
   a. Genetic defect of β cell function due to mutation in various enzymes (maturity onset DM of young)
   b. Genetic defect in insulin processing or insulin action
   c. Diseases of exocrine pancreas
   d. Chronic pancreatitis, pancreatic tumors, post pancreatectomy
   e. Endocrinopathies
   f. Drug and chemical induced (steroid, thiazides)
   g. Infections (congenital rubella, cytomegalovirus)
   h. Gestational diabetes mellitus

Etiology

Defect or derangement in the synthesis, release or action of insulin is key factor for the genesis of this metabolic disorder. Certain environmental factor which alters the action and need of the insulin also results in diabetes mellitus.

Normal Glucose Homeostasis

- **Glucose production** by liver
- **Regulation of glucose level** by insulin and glucagons
- **Utilization of glucose** by tissue

Insulin

Insulin is a major anabolic hormone and it interact with target cells through insulin receptors (Fig. 13.1)

Actions of Insulin

- **On adipose tissue**
  - Increased glucose uptake
  - Increased lipogenesis
  - Decreased lipolysis
- **On striated muscles**
  - Increased glucose uptake
  - Increased glycogen synthesis
  - Increased protein synthesis
- **On liver**
  - Decreased gluconeogenesis

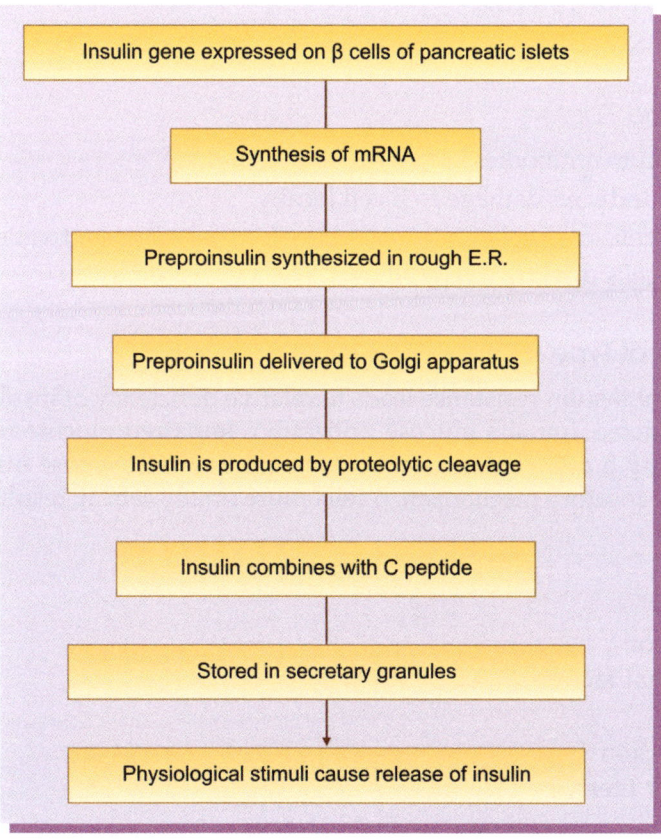

Fig. 13.1: Synthesis and release of insulin

- Increased glycogen synthesis
- Increased lipogenesis

Pathogenesis of Type I Diabetes Mellitus

Complete destruction of β cell mass (at least 80%) leads to absolute insulin deficiency

Causes of Destruction of β Cell Mass

A. Genetic Susceptibility

- 1st order relative are at high risk, identical twins has 70% risk
- 95% shows HLA DR3, HLA DR4 alleles

B. Environmental Factors

- Viral infections
- Chemicals toxins (Strept. toxin, alloxan)
- (?) Bovine milk proteins
- Geographical and seasonal variation

C. Autoimmune Factors

- Islet cell auto antibodies
- Cytokine induced damage to β cell locally
- CD-4 + T cells cause tissue injury through macrophage activation
- CD-8 + T cells directly kill β cell

Pathogenesis of Type II Diabetes Mellitus

Development of insulin resistance leads to relative deficiency of insulin. Receptor and post receptor defect impairs glucose utilization. Impaired glucose utilization results in compensatory β cell hyperplasia. Prolonged impaired glucose utilization leads to failure of compensatory mechanism. β cell failure finally sets in, resulting into diabetes mellitus.

Causes of Development of Insulin Resistance

A. Genetic factor
B. Constitutional factors
- Obesity
- Hypertension
- Sedentary lifestyle

Pathogenesis of maturity onset diabetes mellitus of young (MODY)

Autosomal dominant genetic defect results in defect in β cell function

Clinical Features

Type I Diabetes Mellitus

- Abrupt onset at about 20 years of age
- Present with polydipsia, polyphagia, polyuria and weight loss
- Ketoacidosis may develop

Type II Diabetes Mellitus

- Insidious onset after the age of 40
- Generally asymptomatic, obese
- May complain of weakness and sudden weight loss

Maturity onset Diabetes Mellitus of Young

- Early onset usually before the age of 25
- Not obese, present with three poly's and weight loss

Diagnosis of Diabetes Mellitus

1. Urine glucose test for glycosuria. Benedict's test qualitative test is employed to detect sugar in urine. It is however not specific for sugar. Many reducing substances like vitamin C may give false positive results.
2. Oral glucose tolerance test
   - After overnight fasting a blood sample is drawn for glucose estimation
   - 75 gm glucose dissolved in 300 ml of water is given orally
   - Blood samples are drawn for 2 hours at the interval of half an hour and glucose estimation is done

Interpretation

- Diabetes mellitus
  - Fasting blood glucose >125 mg/dl, 2 hours after glucose load >200 mg/dl
- Impaired fasting glucose
  - Fasting blood glucose >110 mg/dl but <125 mg/dl
  - 2 hours after glucose load >140 mg/dl but less than 200 mg/dl

  Glucose tolerance test is considered to be specific and sensitive test to diagnose diabetes mellitus.

  For the maintenance of anti-diabetic therapy, however only fasting and post-parandial glucose estimation may be quite enough.

  For the screening of diabetes mellitus blood sugar random sample is employed.
3. Glycosylated haemoglobin (HbA1C)

   HbA1C estimation is used to estimate average glycemic state during preceding 3 months. Since dietary variations affect random or fasting and post prandial samples, HbA1C is useful for monitoring management of diabetes mellitus.

4. Insulin assay

Plasma insulin level can be estimated using RIA or ELISA technique, but it is useful for the diagnosis of insulin dependent type I DM.

5. C-peptide assay

C-peptide assay is more sensitive than insulin estimation since its level is not affected by insulin therapy.

Complications of Diabetes Mellitus

Two types of complications are seen in diabetes mellitus depending upon onset

A. Acute metabolic complications
  - Ketoacidosis
  - Hyperosmolar nonketotic coma
  - Hypoglycemia

B. Late systemic complications
  1. **Macrovascular disease** affecting large and medium size arteries. Diabetes mellitus accelerate the process of atherosclerosis leading to increased risk of myocardial infarction, stroke, and lower extremity gangrene.
  2. **Microvascular disease** affects capillaries of retina, kidneys and peripheral nerves resulting in retinopathy, nephropathy and neuropathy.

Pathogenesis of Complications

Persistent hyperglycemia leads to structural functional alteration in cell, tissue and organ system. Severity of complication depends upon the duration and level of hyperglycemia. Two biochemical mechanisms have been implicated for the development of complications.

1. Non-enzymatic Glycosylation

- Formation of irreversible **advanced glycosylation end products** (AGEs) by non enzymatic reaction between intracellular glucose and intra- and extracellular proteins. AGE formation occurs on proteins, lipids, and nucleic acids.
- **Cross-linkage of same proteins**—Cross-linkage between molecules of collagen decreases elasticity predisposes vessel to stress endothelial injury.
- **Non-glycosylated proteins are trapped** by AGE. Trapping of LDL retard its efflux from vessel wall and enhances deposition of cholesterol in intima, thus accelerating atherosclerosis.
- In capillaries albumin bind to glycosylated basement membrane leading to thickening of basement membrane (diabetic microangiopathy) AGE cross-linked proteins are **resistant to proteolytic digestion**.
- Age binds to receptors on many cells and induces biological activities like
  - Induction of monocytic migration
  - Release of cytokines and reactive oxygen metabolites

- Increased permeability
- Procoagulant activity
- Cellular proliferation

2. *Polyol Pathway*

- In some tissues which do not require insulin for glucose transport, high intracellular glucose is metabolized by aldolase reductase to sorbitol.
- Accumulated sorbitol and fructose leads to increased intracellular osmolality and osmotic cell injury.

Morphological Features

a. *Pancreas*

- Reduction in size and number of islets
- Neutrophilic insulitis
- In long-standing cases, amyloid replacement of islets

b. *Vascular System*

- Accelerated atherosclerosis
- Hyaline arteriosclerosis
- Microangiopathy

c. *Kidney*

- Glomerular basement membrane thickening
- Diffuse mesangial sclerosis
- Nodular glomerulosclerosis
- Necrotizing papillitis

d. *Ocular*

- Retinopathy
- Cataract
- Glaucoma

e. *Neuropathy*

Peripheral axonal degeneration and segmental demyelination

f. *Defective Immunity*

- Enhanced susceptibility to infection
- Defect in neutrophilic function

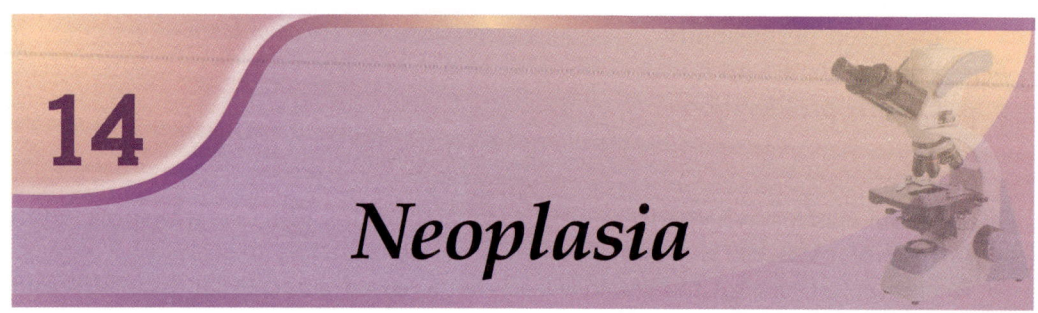

14

Neoplasia

NEOPLASIA (NEW GROWTH OR TUMOR)

It is a mass of tissue formed as the result of Purposeless, Autonomous, Abnormal, and Uncoordinated Proliferation of cells (PAAUP).

Oncology is the subject which deals with the tumors.

Types
1. Benign tumor is a cohesive expansile mass, usually capsulated.
2. Malignant tumors are neoplastic growth of tissue with cellular atypia which invade the surrounding tissue and metastasize to distant places.

Nomenclature

- Benign tumors are designated by adding suffix "oma" to the cell of origin. For example, fibroma, chondroma, adenoma.
- Malignant tumors of epithelial origin are designated as by addition of "carcinoma" to the cell of origin. For example, squamous cell carcinoma, adenocarcinoma, basal cell carcinoma.
- Malignant tumors of mesenchymal origin are designated with the addition of suffix "Sarcoma". For example, osteosarcoma, rhabdomyosarcoma, fibrosarcoma.
- Certain tumors show cells of more than one germ cell origin, are called mixed tumors. For example, pleomorphic salivary adenoma, teratoma.

Choristoma are ectopic rests of normal tissue at abnormal location, for example rests of adrenal in kidney.

Hamartoma: Aberrant differentiation may produce a mass of disorganized but mature tissue indigenous to that site. For example, hamartoma of lung.

Morphological Features of Tumor

Gross Features

- Benign tumors are spherical, ovoid, capsulated firm and of regular shape
- Malignant tumors are irregular, poorly circumscribed, and soft to firm and with secondary changes

Microscopic Features

1. Pattern of Growth

- Pattern of growth suggest cell origin, for example, acini, sheets, cords, gland formation are indicative of tumor of epithelial origin
- Cells when separated by mesenchymal substances like collagen, osteoid material are suggestive tumor of mesenchymal origin

2. Polarity

In benign tumors polarity of cells is maintained, while polarity is lost in malignant tumors

3. Differentiation

- Differentiation is the extent to which cells resemble to mature cell morphologically and functionally. Tumors are designated accordingly as well, moderately or poorly differentiated.
- Benign tumors are composed of completely differentiated tissue.

4. Size and Shape of Cells

- Benign tumors are composed of cells of uniform size and regular shape.
- Malignant tumors show anisocytosis and variation in shape (pleomorphism). Certain tumors appear monotonous because of monoclonal proliferation.

5. Nuclear Features

- Benign cells show uniform size, fine chromatin material and inconspicuous nucleoli. Mitoses are infrequent. Multinucleated giant cells are not seen.
- Malignant cells show anisonucleosis, coarse clumped chromatin and prominent nucleoli with increased nuclear cytoplasmic ratio. Mitotic figures are atypical and frequent. Giant cells are evident in many malignant tumors.

6. Cytoplasmic Features

- Benign tumors show cytoplasm as it appear in mature cell.
- Malignant cells show scanty or abundant cytoplasm with various inclusions.

7. Nuclear Cytoplasmic Ratio

- In benign cells ratio is well maintained.
- In malignant cells nuclear cytoplasmic ratio is high (N/C ratio)

8. Local Invasion in Surrounding Stroma

- Benign tumors show compression phenomenon. Secondary changes like haemorrhage, necrosis, and inflammation are less often.
- Malignant tumors show invasion in surrounding tissue, usually accompanied by secondary changes.

9. Growth Rate

Growth rate of tumor depends on
- Cell division and cell destruction rate
- Non neoplastic element like stroma, secretions, fluid collection

10. Degree of Differentiation

Benign tumors are usually slow growing, while malignant tumors grow very fast

11. Metastasis

Discontinuous tumor mass away from its origin is called metastasis.
- It is the sign of malignancy. Benign tumors do not metastasize
- Majority of malignant tumors metastasize except for few like basal cell carcinoma and glioma which are locally invasive
- Metastasis is used as prognostic marker

Features	Benign tumors	Malignant tumors
Gross features		
Outline	Encapsulated	Ill-defined
Size	Usually small	Usually large
Secondary changes	Less often	Commonly seen
Neighboring tissue	Compressed	Invaded
Microscopic features		
Pattern of growth	Well-differentiated	Mild to poorly differentiated
Polarity	Retained	Lost
Anaplasia	Absent	Present
Mitotic figures	Few, typical	Many, atypical
Nuclear/cytoplasmic ratio	Normal	Increased
Tumor giant cells	Rarely seen	Commonly seen
Other features		
Cytogenetic changes	Rare	Common
Cell function	Maintained	Disturbed
Growth rate	Slow	Fast
Local invasion	Rarely seen	Common
Metastasis	Absent	Present

Pathways of Spread

A. Direct Invasion of Body Cavities and Surface

Tumors penetrate into natural open space directly like pleural, pericardial, and synovial cavity.

B. Lymphatic Spread

- Functional lymphatics are absent in tumor mass. Lymphatics located at the surface are natural route of dissemination

- Predominantly epithelial malignancies prefer this route. Sarcoma may spread through lymphatics but less often
- Drainage of cellular debris and antigens may induce reactive changes in regional lymph nodes
- Sentinel lymph node is first node in regional lymphatic chain to get enlarged by metastasis

C. Haematogenous Spread

- Preferably sarcoma adopts this route for metastasis. Carcinoma may spread but less frequently
- Arteries are thick, therefore, metastasis occurs mainly through veins. All portal blood flows through liver and all vena cava blood through lungs, therefore liver and lungs are most frequent sites of haematogenous spread. Malignancies adjacent to vertebral column like thyroid and prostate metastasize to vertebrae through paravertebral plexus

Mechanism of Metastasis

- A subpopulation of proliferating clone of malignant cells emerges with biological characteristics favoring metastasis
- New blood vessels develop with endothelial gaps which are in direct contact with metastasizing subpopulation
- Cells enter the vascular channels or lymphatics and reach to distant vascular bed or lymph node and proliferate to form metastatic mass

A. Attachment of Tumor Cell to Extracellular Matrix (ECM)

Tumor cells bear increased number of receptors for laminin and fibronectin. Dyscohesive masses of tumor cells get attached to ECM proteins through receptors. ECM loses integrins.

B. Degradation of ECM

Dissolution of basement membrane of tumor, vessels and interstitium takes place by
- Increased metalloproteinase expression on tumors cell
- Increased proteases
- Decreased inhibitors of metalloproteinase (TIMP)

C. Entrance of Tumor Cells in Vessel Lumen

It is influenced by following factors:
- Autocrine motility factors (AMF) stimulate receptor mediated motility of tumor cells
- Cleavage products of matrix induce chemotaxis of tumor cells, promote growth and neoangiogenesis

D. *Growth of Tumor Cells*

Elaboration of growth factors promotes growth and survival of metastatic tumor deposit at a distant new place.

Epidemiology of Neoplasia

Factors influencing neoplastic proliferation are:

1. *Familial and Genetic Factors*

Cancer with a high frequency of occurrence in families is called familial cancers. Characteristic features are
• Onset is at an early age
• Multiple malignancies are seen in a single individual
• No definite pattern of transmission is identified
   For example, carcinoma breast, colon, uterus, stomach and sarcomas.

Mechanism of Development of Neoplasm in Families

a. Autosomal dominant inherited cancer syndrome
   Autosomal dominant mutant gene with point mutation in one allele of tumor suppression gene is transmitted to offspring. Defect in second allele occur generally as a consequence of deletion or recombination. For example
   1. Retinoblastoma (Rb gene): 40% of retinoblastoma is seen in families. Carrier of mutant gene is at high risk of development of retinoblastoma and second cancer like, osteosarcoma.
   2. Familial polyposis coli: Autosomal dominant inheritance, polypoid adenoma is present at birth and polyposis coli develop by the age of 60.
   3. MEN syndrome
      MEN I—Adenomas of pituitary, parathyroid and pancreas
      MEN II—Medullary carcinoma of thyroid, pheochromocytoma and parathyroid tumor
   4. Neurofibromatosis or von Recklinghausen's disease: Autosomal dominant disease, manifesting as neurofibromatosis and café au lait spots
b. Defective DNA repair syndrome
   Four types of DNA repair genes
   1. Mismatch repair gene
   2. Base excision gene
   3. Nucleotide excision gene
   4. Double-strand break repair gene
   Defect in DNA repair genes produce DNA instability which leads to neoplasm development. For example, xeroderma pigmentosa is an autosomal recessive disorder with sensitivity to UV light and predisposes to basal cell carcinoma, squamous cell carcinoma and melanoma.

2. *Racial and Geographical Factors*

In white Europeans commonly carcinoma of skin, penis, cervix and liver are seen. Japanese are more likely to suffer from carcinoma stomach. Indians show more incidence of oral and GIT cancers, carcinoma of cervix and breast.

3. *Environmental and Cultural Factors*

Diet, habits, customs and cultural factors has been found to be associated with specific cancers. For example
- Oral cancers, carcinoma of larynx, lung, pancreas and urinary bladder are commonly seen in tobacco chewer and cigarette/bidi smokers
- Oropharyngeal cancers, esophageal and liver cancers are common in alcoholics
- Industrial chemicals and environmental pollutants are associated with cancers of respiratory tract, GIT and skin. For example, arsenic, asbestos, benzene, vinyl chloride, beta naphthylamine, etc.
- Dietary factors like obesity, deficiency of vitamin A, tocopherol, selenium and zinc may predispose to carcinoma.

4. *Age and Sex*

- Cancers are commonly observed in old age
- Certain tumors of germ cell origin are common in childhood age
- Incidence of malignancy is more in male than female
- Breast, thyroid and gall bladder carcinoma are more common in female
- Lung cancer is common in male

5. *Premalignant Conditions*

- Many benign lesions may predispose to development of malignancy for example. Multiple adenoma colon may get converted into adenocarcinoma. Neuro-fibromatosis may turn into sarcoma.
- Carcinoma *in situ* may progress to carcinoma. For example, *in situ* changes of cervix, Bowen's disease of penis, solar keratosis and leukoplakia of skin.
- Long-standing inflammatory lesion may induce malignant changes, for example ulcerative colitis, cirrhosis, chronic bronchitis, chronic irritation by loose dentures.

CARCINOGENESIS

The process of development of neoplastic lesion is known as carcinogenesis. Carcinogens which induce tumor formation are

1. Chemical Carcinogens

Induction of cancer depends on
- Dose, duration and mode of administration of chemicals
- Susceptibility of individual
- Associated predisposing conditions

A. Initiation

Irreversible changes brought about in cells by initiator chemicals acting for long duration in small doses or over a short time in large doses. Various initiator chemicals are:

1. Directly Acting Carcinogens

a. Alkylating agents
- Anticancer drugs like cyclophosphamide, chlorambucil, busulfan, malphalan
- Beta propiolactone
- Dimethyl sulphate
- Diepoxybutane

b. Acylating agents
- 1-acetyl imidazole
- Dimethylcarbamoyl chloride

2. Indirectly Acting (Procarcinogens)

a. Polycyclic aromatic hydrocarbons found in tobacco, smoke, fossil fuel, tar, mineral oil, soot smoked animal food can cause lung, skin, oral cancer and sarcoma
- Anthracenes
- Banzopyrene
- Methylcholanthrene

b. Aromatic amines and azo dyes can cause bladder carcinoma, hepatocellular carcinoma
- Betanaphthylamine
- Banzidine
- Butter yellow, scarlet red

c. Naturally occurring products are also responsible for tumor formation like
- Aflatoxin
- Cycasin
- Safrole
- Betelnut

d. Miscellaneous
- Nitrosamine and amides cause gastric carcinoma
- Vinyl chloride monomer cause angiocarcinoma of liver
- Asbestos can cause bronchogenic carcinoma, mesothelioma
- Metal (nickel, lead, cobalt, chromium) cause epidermal hyperplasia and basal cell carcinoma
- Insecticide, fungicide, polychlorinated biphenyls

B. *Promotion*

Altered cell express monoclonal proliferation in response to certain chemical promoters. These promoter chemicals are:

- Phenol
- Phenobarbitals
- Phorbol esters
- Hormones
- Saccharine

Mechanism of Chemical Carcinogenesis

I. *Metabolic Activation of Chemical Carcinogens*

Procarcinogens are converted into electron deficient carcinogens in endoplasmic reticulum of hepatocytes by mono oxygenase of cytochrome P450.

II. *Mutagenesis*

Electron deficient carcinogen bounds to electron rich part of cell (DNA, RNA and proteins). It causes permanent DNA damage. Unrepaired damage is converted into permanent damage. Permanent damage is transmitted to progeny after proliferation of cell.

III. *Promotion*

Altered progeny undergo monoclonal proliferation by promoter carcinogens, leading to development of neoplastic cell.

2. Physical Carcinogens

a. Radiation may induce carcinogenesis by its ionizing properties resulting in damage to DNA.
   - Ultraviolet rays on long-term exposure may leads to cancer at exposed part. Albino and fair skin persons are more prone to develop skin cancers.
   - Ionizing radiations like α, β, and γ radiation, X-rays induces mutation and damage DNA leading to leukaemia, skin, breast and thyroid cancers.
     - Radium watch workers developed lip cancer and osteosarcoma
     - Survivors of atomic bomb blast developed leukaemia and other cancers

b. Non-radiation physical carcinogens like mechanical friction may lead to carcinoma. For example
   - Adenocarcinoma of gallbladder due to gallstones
   - Urinary bladder malignancies due to bladder calculi
   - Carcinoma oral cavity due to loose dentures

3. Hormonal Carcinogens

a. Organ and tissue which undergo proliferation by hormone stimulation may induce neoplastic changes by excessive hormone level. For example
   - Women receiving estrogen therapy are at increased risk of endometrial carcinoma
   - Contraceptive pills taken for long duration may induce benign tumors of liver
b. Certain tumors are hormone dependent and tumor regression occur on removal of hormonal stimulus. For example
   - Prostatic carcinoma responds to estrogen therapy
   - Breast carcinoma regress with oophorectomy
   - Thyroid cancer may regress by administration of thyroxin that suppresses TSH

4. Biologic Carcinogens

Mainly virus cause neoplastic changes; such virus is known as oncogenic virus.

A. Oncogenic DNA virus

These are
- HPV—Human papillomavirus
- EBV—Epstein-Barr virus
- HBV—Hepatitis B virus
- KSHV—Kaposi's sarcoma herpes virus

Genome of oncogenic virus is integrated with host genome and forms a stable association. HPV genome is present in nonintegrated form in benign lesions.

1. HPV (Human Papillomavirus)

- More than 100 subtypes are found.
- Subtype 1, 2, 4, and 7 cause benign squamous papilloma.
- HPV subtype 16, 18, 31, 33, 35, and 51 have been found to be associated with squamous cell carcinoma.
- HPV subtype 6 and 11 cause genital lesions with low malignant potential.

Mechanism
- HPV E6 and E7 block p53 and Rb cell cycle suppression pathway.
- E6 protein of high risk HPV type forms a complex with p53 and enhances its degradation. Increased degradation of p53 causes block in apoptosis.
- E7 from high risk type binds to Rb protein, releasing sequestrated E2F from the Rb-E2F complex, triggering the entry of cells in the S phase.
- E6 and E7 from low risk type has lower affinity for p53 and Rb protein.

2. EBV (Epstein-Barr Virus)

It is associated with pathogenesis of
- Burkitt's lymphoma

- B cell lymphoma
- Hodgkin's lymphoma
- Nasopharyngeal carcinoma

Mechanism

- EBV gets attached to cells of oropharynx and B lymphocytes by CD-21. Linear genome of EBV gets encircled to form episome in B cells
- Normal immune system keep infected cell inactive
- Deficient immune system leads to activation of infected cell by CD-40, which promotes B cell survival and proliferation
- Rapidly dividing cells are at risk of development of mutations
- Activation of MYC gene with Ig gene leads to uncontrolled proliferation

3. HBV (Hepatitis B Virus)

- 70 to 80% of hepatocellular carcinoma is because of HBV and HCV
- HBV cause chronic liver disease and regeneration hyperplasia hence has increased poll of cycling cells, which are at risk of genetic changes

Mechanism

- HBV encodes a regulatory element called HBX protein which disrupts normal growth control of infected liver cells by
  - Transcriptional activation of insulin like growth factor I and II
  - Binds to p53 and interferes with its growth suppressing activities

4. HSV (Herpes Simplex Virus)

It causes Kaposi's sarcoma, B cell lymphoma

Mechanism

HSV 8 infects the host macrophages and primitive mesenchymal cells which differentiate into endothelial cells

B. Oncogenic RNA Virus

RNA viruses contain reverse transcriptase which converts viral RNA into DNA. Transcripted DNA is incorporated in host DNA.

HTLV

- It has been associated with T cell lymphoma leukaemia endemic in Japan and Caribbean basin.
- HTLV has tropism for CD-4 + T cells. Infected T cells are transmitted by sexual contact, blood products and breast feeding.

Mechanism

HTLV contain TAX gene which activate several host genes involved in proliferation and differentiation of T cells and interference with DNA repair.

C. Bacterial Carcinogenesis

H. pylori

- *H. pylori* have been found in 90% cases of gastritis and 20–30% cases of gastric carcinoma
- It may be associated with gastric carcinoma and gastric lymphoma
- It possess CagA and VacV virulence associated genes
- Active B cell proliferation predispose to genetic abnormality

5. Molecular Genes (Oncogenes)

A. Excessive and Autonomous Growth

- Genes that promotes autonomous cell growth in cancer are called oncogenes
- Proto-oncogenes are physiological regulators of cell proliferation and differentiation
- Oncogenes are mutated form of normal proto-oncogenes

Oncogenes differ from proto-oncogenes

- By the presence of mutation in structure of the gene
- Oncogenes have ability to promote cell growth in the absence of normal mitogens
- Over expression of oncogenes lead to autonomous and excessive proliferation

Activation of oncogenes occur by

i. Point mutation and deletion, for example
   - RAS oncogene in carcinoma of urinary bladder and pancreas
ii. Chromosomal translocation, for example
   - Philadelphia chromosome seen in chronic myeloid leukaemia (translocation of C-ABL proto-oncogene from chromosome 9 to chromosome 22)
   - In Burkitt's lymphoma translocation of CMYC proto-oncogene from chromosome 8 to 14 is seen.
iii. Gene amplification, for example
   - In neuroblastoma nMYC
   - In breast and ovarian carcinoma ERB-B2

B. Refractoriness to Growth Inhibition (Growth suppressing antioncogenes)

Deficiency of antioncogenes or mutated antioncogenes act as growth promoter and leads to neoplastic transformation

- In retinoblastoma Rb and p53 gene situated on chromosome 13q14 are either absent or defective.
- In Wilm's tumor, WT-1 gene which prevent neoplastic proliferation in embryonic kidney is absent or defective.
- BRCA1 gene located on the long arm of chromosome 17 is involved in DNA repair and regulation of transcription. Variation in BRCA1 gene has been linked to breast, ovarian and prostatic carcinoma.

- BRCA2 is located on long arm of chromosome 13, and is essential for DNA repair. Abnormality of BRCA2 cause increased risk of carcinoma breast, ovaries, prostate, pancreas and melanoma.

C. Mutator Gene

Mutator genes are caretaker genes for integrity of genetic material, when mutation occur in mutator gene, it loses surveillance function and render DNA susceptible to mutations. For example
- Hereditary non polyposis colonic carcinoma
- Ataxia telangiectasia has ATM gene (mutated gene)

Theories of Carcinogenesis

1. Genetic Theory

Basic mechanism involved is alteration in DNA that leads to neoplastic transformation. Evidences in the favor of theory are
- Physical and chemical agents bring about mutation
- Cell is unable to repair the DNA damage caused by UV rays, in xeroderma pigmentosum
- Viral DNA is integrated in host DNA in malignancies induced by oncogenic virus
- Specific chromosomal abnormality is associated with certain malignancy like Philadelphia chromosomes in chronic myeloid leukaemia
- Activation of oncogene or suppression of antioncogene, in retinoblastoma

2. Epigenetic Theory

Carcinogenic agents act on activators and suppressors of genes and not on the genes resulting in abnormal expression of gene. This theory is less well supported.

3. The Multistep Theory (Fig. 14.1)

Carcinogenesis is a multistep process. For example
- In chemical carcinogenesis two steps are there: initiator and promoters
- Most cancers arise after several mutations which have been acquired in proper sequence
- Many tumors arise from combination of activation of growth promoting oncogenes and inactivation of growth suppressing antioncogenes
- In some cases initial step is dysplasia that progresses to invasive carcinoma
  This theory is well accepted and well documented *in vivo* and *in vitro* experiments.

4. Immunosurveillance Theory

Immunocompetent individual destroys the developing tumor cells while immuno-incompetent individual fails to do so. Evidences in support are:
- High incidences of cancers in immunodeficient individuals
- Most cancers occur in old ages when immune responses are weak

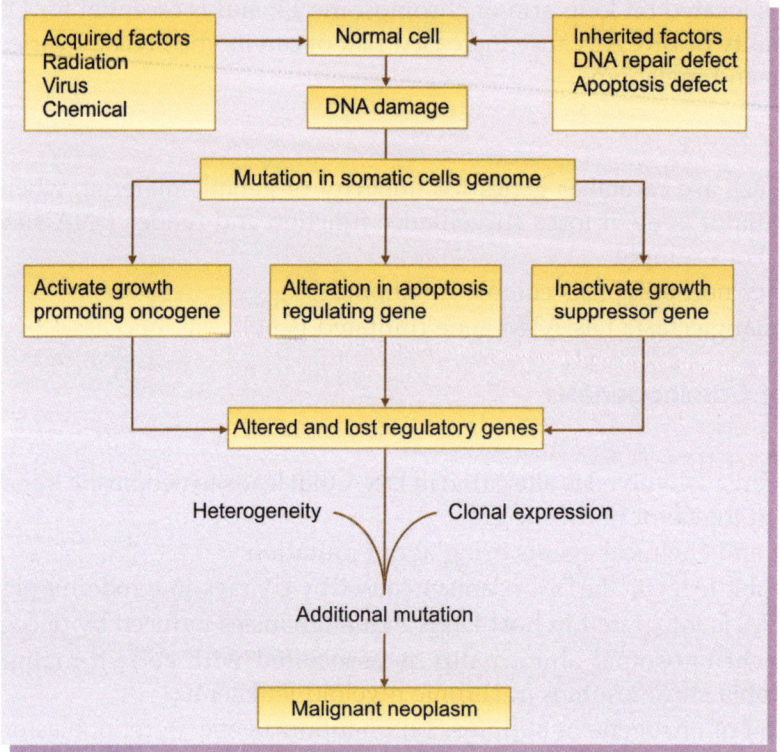

Fig. 14.1: Schematic diagram of malignant transformation

- In experiments high level of immune complexes are seen during tumor induction which decline afterward
- Certain tumors show lymphocytic infiltration in stroma with better prognosis, for example medullary carcinoma of breast and seminoma testis
- Some tumors disappear spontaneously from primary site due to good immune attack by the host and reappear as metastasis subsequently, for example malignant melanoma

5. *Monoclonal Hypothesis*

Most cancers arise from single clone of transformed cells, supported by following examples
- Multiple myeloma produces single type of immunoglobulin
- Many haematopoietic malignancies show same surface markers over transformed cells
- In heterozygous G6PD women, the leiomyoma produced contain either of genotype of G6PD and not both, suggest tumor derived from single progenitor cell

Clinical Features

A. Local Symptoms

Compression, obstruction, because of tumor mass
Destruction, infarction, ulceration in the surrounding tissue

B. General Symptoms

1. Advanced disseminated terminally ill patient show asthenia, anorexia, cachexia.
2. Fever of unexplained origin.

C. Paraneoplastic Syndrome

These are symptom complex in patients with advanced cancer which cannot be assigned to metastasis or hormone released by tumor cells. It is of clinical significance because it may appear some times at earlier stage. It may be classified as

1. Endocrinopathies

   Ectopic hormone or hormone like substances produced by cells of non endocrine origin. For example

   - Small cell carcinoma of lung, pancreatic carcinoma; neural tumors produce ACTH or ACTH like substances resulting in Cushing's syndrome
   - Squamous cell carcinoma of lung, carcinoma breast, kidney, and ovaries produce parathormone or related hormone TNF-α, TNF-β, IL-1 causing hypercalcaemia
   - Gastric and bronchial carcinoid syndromes are produced by elaboration of serotonin and bradykinin by bronchial adenoma, pancreatic carcinoma and gastric carcinoma

2. Nerve and muscle syndrome
   - Immunologically mediated myasthenia gravis in bronchogenic carcinoma
   - Disorders of central and peripheral nervous system seen in breast carcinoma

3. Dermatological disorders
   - Acanthosis nigricans can be seen in carcinoma of lung, uterus, and stomach
   - Dermatomyositis may be seen in bronchogenic and breast carcinoma

4. Vascular and haematological changes
   - Tumor products usually mucin may activate clotting factors causing thrombosis in pancreatic and bronchogenic carcinoma
   - Nonbacterial thrombotic endocarditis is seen in advanced cancers
   - Anaemia may develop in association with thymic neoplasm

5. Bone and tissue changes

   Hypertrophic osteoarthropathy and clubbing may be seen in bronchogenic carcinoma

Laboratory Diagnosis of Cancer

A. *Cytology*

It is good screening procedure of malignancy

1. Fine needle aspiration cytology (FNAC)
   - Material received from tumor mass by needle aspiration directly or under USG guide is spread over glass slide, stained and examined under the microscopic for the evidence of malignancy.
2. Exfoliative cytology
   - Pap smear—Material is obtained from vagina and cervix. Smears are examined after staining for the evidence of malignancy (Fig. 14.2).
   - Body fluid cytology—Pleural, peritoneal, pericardial, bronchial fluid is examined for the evidence of malignancy.
   - Urine, sputum CSF and gastric secretions are examined for the evidence of malignancy.

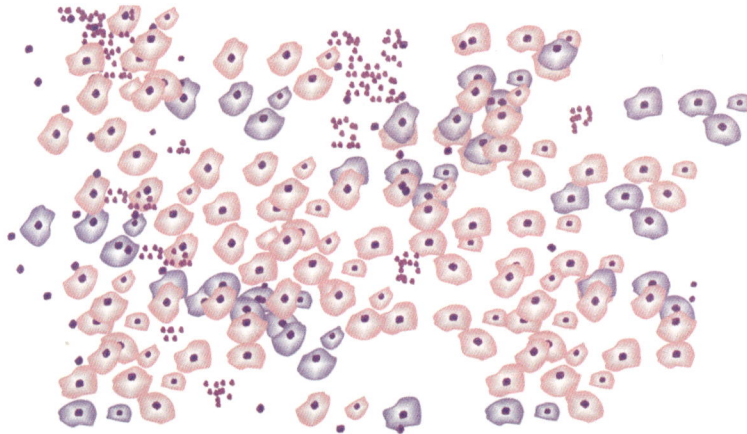

Fig. 14.2: Pap smear

B. *Histopathology*

- Specimens are processed for thin sectioning and histological sections are examined for the evidence of malignancy. It is gold standard procedure for malignancy diagnosis (Fig. 14.3).

C. *Histochemistry/Cytochemistry*

- These are diagnostic tools for tumor classification and identification of cell origin. For example, PAS stain used for basement membrane identification
- Reticulin stain for reticulin fiber pattern
- Mucicarmine for mucin identification
- Sudan black for fat identification

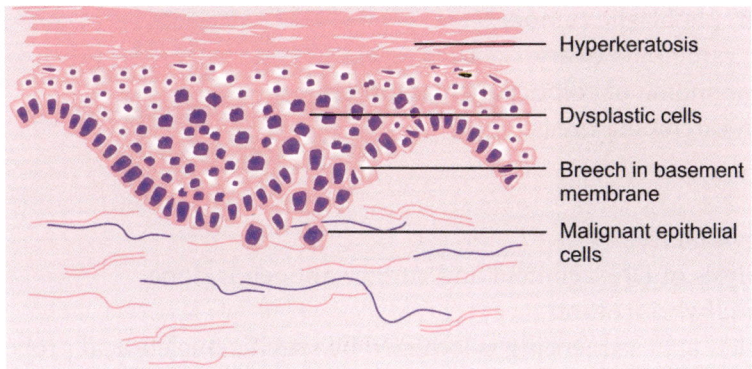

Hyperkeratosis

Dysplastic cells

Breech in basement membrane

Malignant epithelial cells

Fig. 14.3: Carcinoma *is situ* with microinvasion

D. *Immunohistochemistry*

- Immunological method is used to recognize a cell based on identification of specific antigen present over surface. Specific antibodies are prepared by hybridoma technique and labeled with enzymes to activate specific fluorochromes.
- It is used in identification of poorly differentiated or undifferentiated tumors.
- Keratin marker (carcinoma, mesothelioma, germ cell tumor), vimentin marker (sarcoma, melanoma, lymphoma), desmin marker (myogenic tumor).
- Specifying type of leukaemia, lymphoma.
- Determination of origin of metastatic tumors.
- It is also used to identify prognostic markers, for example, ER, PR and HER nu in breast carcinoma.

E. *Electron Microscopy*

It is used for confirmation of tumor typing and classification by
- Presence of type of cell junction
- Presence of microvilli
- Features of nucleus and nuclear membrane
- Nucleolar features
- Cytoplasmic organelles
- Presence of dense bodies in cytoplasm

F. *Tumor Markers*

These are substances found in blood, fluid, urine, or tissue which are associated with tumor. These are used for diagnosis and prognostic purpose, for example
- AFP in hepatocellular carcinoma, germ cell tumors
- PSA in prostatic carcinoma

- HCG in trophoblastic tumors
- Ca-125 in carcinoma ovary
- CEA in carcinoma of colon, pancreas, breast
- Ca-15.3 in carcinoma breast

G. Newer Tests

1. Flow cytometry
    - Analysis of DNA content and surface antigen is done
    - *In situ* hybridization
    - Nucleic acid sequencing is localized by specific nucleic acid probes directly in the cell
2. Other molecular techniques
    - Analysis of molecular cytogenetics
    - Mutational analysis
    - Antigen receptor gene rearrangement
    - Study of oncogenic viruses

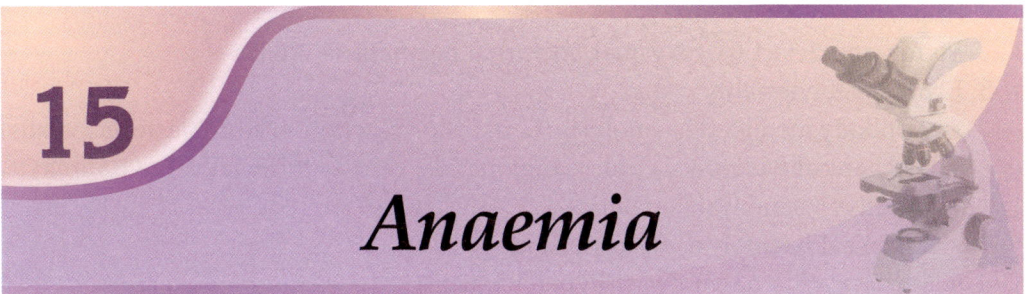

15

Anaemia

DEFINITION

Anaemia is defined as reduction in the oxygen carrying capacity of the blood. It is designated as reduction in packed cell volume (PCV) and reduction in haemoglobin content (Hb) below normal limits.

Normal haemoglobin: 12–16 gm/dl

Classification

Etiological Classification

1. Anaemia due to blood loss
   a. Acute loss
      • Trauma, postpartum bleeding, major surgery
   b. Chronic blood loss
      • Bleeding through GIT (hemorrhoids, peptic ulcer, carcinoma, worms)
      • Genitourinary tract (menstrual disorders, calculi)
2. Impaired red cell production
   • Nutritional deficiency (iron, vitamin B_{12}, folic acid)
   • Bone marrow invasion (leukaemia, myelofibrosis, secondary carcinoma)
   • Bone marrow failure (hypoplastic, aplastic anaemia)
   • Endocrine deficiency (hypothyroidism, hypoadrenalism, hypopituitarism)
   • Renal and hepatic diseases
   • Chronic infective and inflammatory diseases
   • Sideroblastic anaemia
3. Excessive destruction of red cells
   A. Intrinsic abnormality in RBCs
      Genetic disorder
      • Membrane defect (spherocytosis, ovalocytosis)
      • Metabolic defect (G6PD deficiency, PK deficiency)
      • Dyserythropoietic defect (thalassemia, sickle cell anaemia)

Acquired

Membrane defect (paroxysmal nocturnal haematuria, PNH)

B. Extrinsic abnormality

- Antibody mediated haemolysis (transfusion reaction, erythroblastosis foetalis)
- Mechanical haemolysis (microangiopathic, cardiac artificial valve trauma)
- Infective haemolysis (malaria)
- Chemical haemolysis (lead poisoning)
- Sequestration haemolysis (hypersplenism)

Morphological Classification

1. Microcytic anaemia: Iron deficiency anaemia
2. Macrocytic anaemia: Megaloblastic anaemia, haemorrhage
3. Normocytic anaemia: Aplastic anaemia

Clinical Features of Anaemia

General Symptoms

- Fatigue, lassitude, dyspnoea, palpitation, dizziness, syncope, tinnitus, vertigo
- Irritability, sleep disturbances, lack of concentration, headache, paresthesia
- Anorexia, nausea, bowel disturbances, amenorrhoea, polymenorrhoea

Signs of Anaemia

- Skin and mucus membrane, nails, conjunctiva appear pale white
- Tachycardia with increased pulse pressure, ejection systolic murmur
- Pedal edema, puffiness over face, cardiac dilatation

IRON DEFICIENCY ANAEMIA

Iron deficiency anaemia is most common type of anaemia seen in clinical practice.

Etiology

1. Pathological blood loss

   All types of bleeding from GIT, GUT and epistaxis leads to loss of iron
2. Increased physiological demand

   Growing children, pregnancy demand more iron supply
3. Inadequate intake
   - Nutritional deficiency
   - Diet deficient of iron sources, anorexia, poor bioavailability of iron
   - Impairment in absorption and utilization of iron in gastrectomy, tropical sprue, celiac disease, chronic diarrhoea

Iron Metabolism

Dietary iron is available from two sources
a. Haem iron (animal source iron is readily absorbed)
b. Non haem iron (vegetables iron is poorly absorbed)

Iron Statistics

- Total body iron   3–5 g
- Iron in haemoglobin   2.3 g
- Stored tissue iron (available iron)   1.0 g
- Essential iron present in myoglobin
  and enzymes (non available iron)   0.5 g
- Non haem iron is transported in portal circulation with the help of DMT1 (metal transporter), ferro protein (transporter) and hephaestin (iron oxide).
- Haem iron enters through mucosa unchanged, and then iron is released by enzyme haem oxygenase with in the cell. Ferritin containing cells are exfoliated and lost in faeces.
- Normal loss of iron in faeces, urine, and sweat is 0.5–1 mg per day
- Iron lost in menses is 0.5–1 mg per cycle

Steps of Developments of Iron Deficiency Anaemia

1. Stored iron is depleted
2. Iron deficient erythropoiesis
3. Frank iron deficiency anaemia

Clinical Features

Symptoms due to anaemia
Lassitude, weakness, fatigue, dyspnoea, palpitation, pallor skin and mucus membrane

Symptoms due to epithelial changes (induced by hypoxia)
- Nails— thin lusterless, brittle, ridging and flattening, koilonychia
- Tongue—atrophy of papillae, shiny or glazed tongue, glossitis, angular stomatitis

Laboratory Findings

Complete blood cell count
- Haemoglobin   decreased
- Total RBC count   decreased
- RBC indices (MCV, MCH, and MCHC)   low

  Peripheral blood smear examination reveals microcytosis, hypochromasia (Fig. 15.1)
  - Increased RDW (Red cell distribution width) indicating anisocytosis, poikilocytosis
  - Platelets and WBC are normal
  - Reticulocyte count is normal or decreased

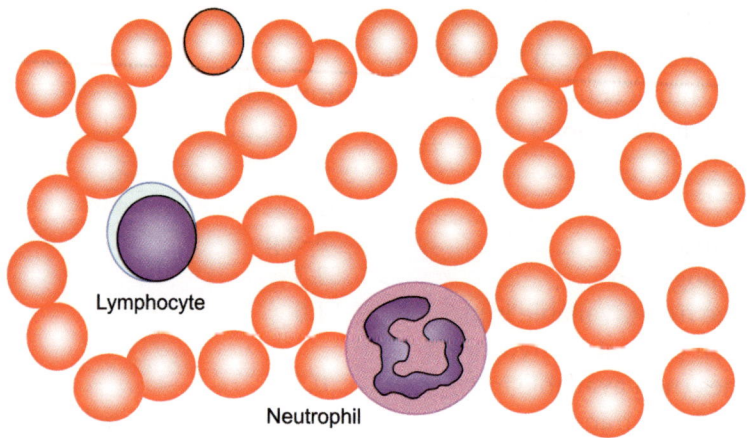

Fig. 15.1: Microcytic hypochromic anaemia

Bone marrow shows erythroid hyperplasia with depleted iron stores

Biochemical profile
- Serum iron   low (normal 50–180 mg/dl)
- Serum ferritin   low (normal 20–300 microgram /L)
- Total iron binding capacity   high (normal 2.5–4 mg /L)
- Transferrin saturation   low (normal 33%)

MEGALOBLASTIC ANAEMIA

Megaloblastic anaemia results from asynchrony between nuclear and cytoplasmic maturation. It is a type of macrocytic anaemia due to impaired DNA synthesis, RNA synthesis remains unaffected.

Megaloblastic Erythropoiesis

It is the process of red cell synthesis in which nuclear maturation lags behind the cytoplasmic maturation. It results in larger volume of cytoplasm of megaloblastic erythroid series cells, hence the name.

Causes of Megaloblastic Anaemia

1. Deficiency of vitamin B_{12}
   - Decreased intake of vitamin B_{12} in diet, vegetarian diet (deficient in vitamin B_{12})
   - Impaired absorption due to intrinsic factor deficiency (pernicious anaemia), mal absorption states, ileal resection, diffuse intestinal disease, fish tapeworm infection
   - Increased requirement in pregnancy, hyperthyroidism, disseminated cancer

2. Deficiency of folic acid
   - Decreased intake due to inadequate diet, alcohol, breast mild (deficient in folate)
   - Impaired absorption in malabsorption states, intrinsic intestinal disease, anticonvulsant and contraceptive drugs
   - Increased requirement in pregnancy, infancy, disseminated cancer
   - Impaired utilization by folic acid antagonists
3. Other causes
   - Metabolic inhibitors like mercaptopurines, fluorouracil
   - Pyridoxine and thiamine deficiency
   - Acute erythroleukaemia

Vitamin B$_{12}$ statistics
- Daily requirement   2–4 microgram
- Daily intake   5–30 microgram
- Body store   2–5 mg (enough for 2–4 years)

Mechanism of Absorption of Vitamin B$_{12}$ (Fig. 15.2)

- Vitamin B$_{12}$ remains attached to protein in food and released in stomach by proteolysis (by pepsin)
- B$_{12}$ combines with R protein and carried to duodenum where R binder is cleaved by pancreatic enzymes
- In duodenum B$_{12}$ combines with intrinsic factor (IF) secreted by parietal cell of stomach
- In ileum B$_{12}$-IF complex binds to receptor on ileal mucosa in the presence of calcium. B$_{12}$ is released in portal blood where it combines with transcobalamin II (TCII) and distributed to tissues
- Transport form of B$_{12}$ is called methylcobalamin
- Storage form is called adenosylcobalamin

Mechanism of Folic Acid Absorption

- In food it exits in poly glutamate form
- Folate is absorbed in proximal jejunum and ileum, mechanism is unclear
- Conjugases in ileal brush border breaks polyglutamate into monoglutamate for absorption
- In plasma it circulates as N 5-methyl tetrahydrofolate free or bound to albumin
- Folic acid is stored in liver in polyglutamate form

Folic acid statistics
- Daily requirement   100–200 microgram
- Daily intake   100–500 microgram
- Body store   5–20 mg (enough for 4 months)

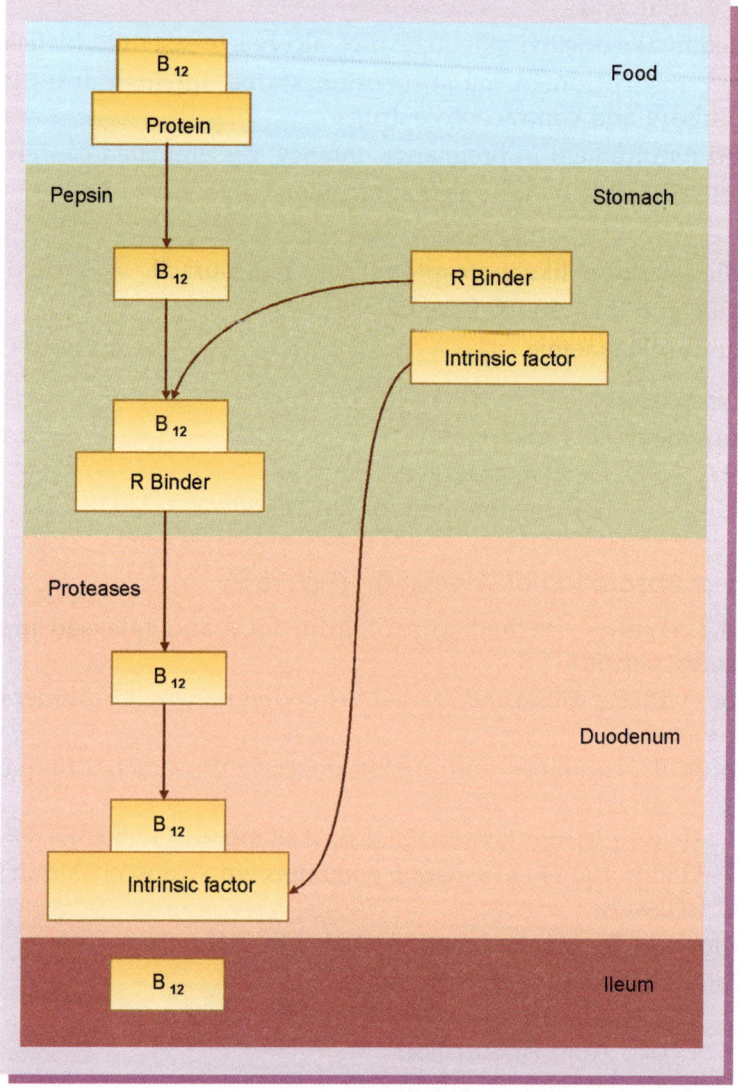

Fig. 15.2: Absorption of vitamin B_{12}

Interaction of Vitamin B_{12} and Folic Acid in DNA Synthesis (Fig. 15.3)

- N5 methyl FH_4 gives methyl group to homocysteine and form methionin. This reaction requires vitamin B_{12}.
- N5 FH_4 is reconjugated to form N5,10 methylene FH_4, which is used for conversion of dUMP (uridine monophosphate) to dTMP (thymidine monophosphate).
- dTMP is used in DNA synthesis.

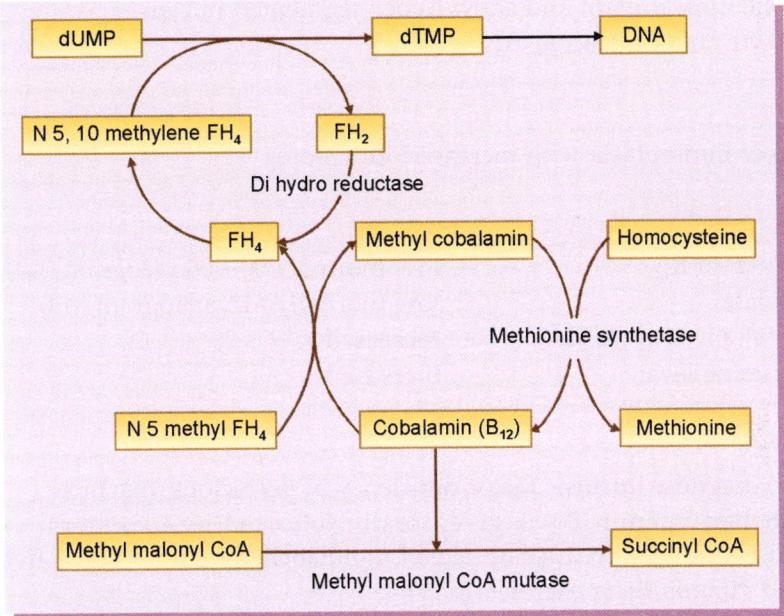

Fig. 15.3: Interaction of vitamin B$_{12}$ and folic acid in DNA synthesis

Clinical Features

1. Symptoms due to anaemia: Lassitude, weakness, fatigue, dyspnoea, palpitation, pallor skin and mucus membrane
2. Symptoms due to degenerative neural changes: Subacute combined myelin degeneration of posterior and lateral tract of spinal cord
3. Symptoms due to epithelial changes: Glossitis

Folic acid deficiency shows all above features except glossitis.

Laboratory Diagnosis

Complete Blood Cell count

- Haemoglobin   Decreased
- Total RBC count   Decreased
- RBC indices (MCV)   Increased
            (MCH)   Decreased

Peripheral Blood Smear (Fig. 15.4)

- Macro-ovalocytosis, hypochromasia
- Increased RDW (Red cell distribution width) indicating anisocytosis poikilocytosis, Howell-Jolly bodies and Cabot's ring bodies may be seen
- Platelets may be reduced with bizarre forms

- Neutrophil appear giant and show hyper segmented nuclei.
- Reticulocyte count is decreased.

Bone Marrow

Megaloblastic hyperplasia with increased iron stores

Biochemical Profile

- Serum vitamin B_{12} low (normal 200–900 picogram/ml)
- Serum folate   low (normal 6–12 nanogram/ml)
- Methylmalonic acid (MMA)   Increased
- Homocysteine level   Increased

Schilling Test

It is used to diagnose intrinsic factor deficiency in pernicious anaemia.
- Radiolabelled vitamin B_{12} is given orally followed by parenteral vitamin B_{12} (1 mg) in 1–6 hours to reduce uptake of radiolabelled vitamin B_{12} by liver
- Absorbed vitamin B_{12} is excreted in urine
- 24 hours urine is collected and amount of radiolabelled vitamin B_{12} excreted is measured
- If more than 9% of dose given orally appears in urine, it is suggestive of normal absorption of vitamin B_{12}
- If radiolabelled vitamin B_{12} in urine is less than 9%, it is suggestive of inadequate vitamin B_{12} absorption
- If absorption improves by giving intrinsic factor, it suggests deficiency of intrinsic factor

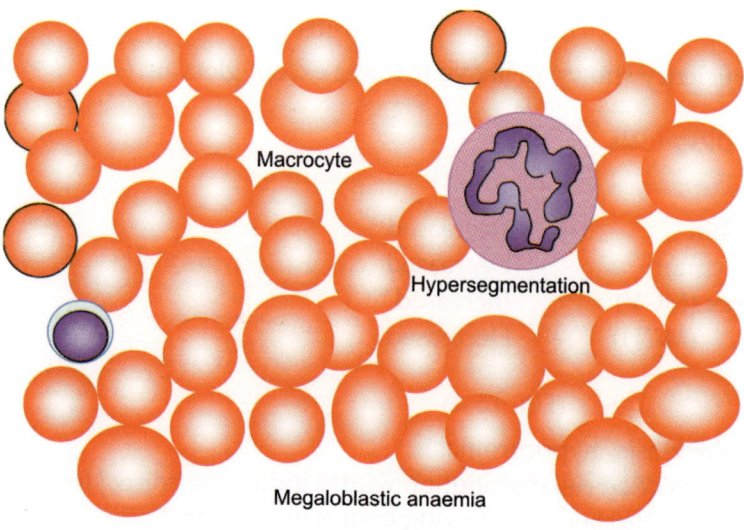

Macrocyte

Hypersegmentation

Megaloblastic anaemia

Fig. 15.4: Megaloblastic anaemia

HAEMOLYTIC ANAEMIA

Haemolytic anaemia is characterized by reduced lifespan of red cells, accumulation of products of hemoglobin catabolism and increased erythropoiesis in marrow (Fig. 15.5).

A. Evidence of increased extravascular haemolysis

- Serum bilirubin (unconjugated) Increased
- Fecal stercobilinogen   Increased
- Urine urobilinogen   Increased
- Plasma LDH   Increased

B. Evidence of increased intravascular haemolysis

- Serum haptoglobin and hemopexin reduced or absent
- Haemoglobinaemia, haemoglobinuria, methalbuminaemia, haemosiderinuria
- Jaundice

C. Evidence of compensatory erythroid hyperplasia

- Reticulocyte count increased
- Microcytosis, polychromasia
- Erythroid hyperplasia in bone marrow

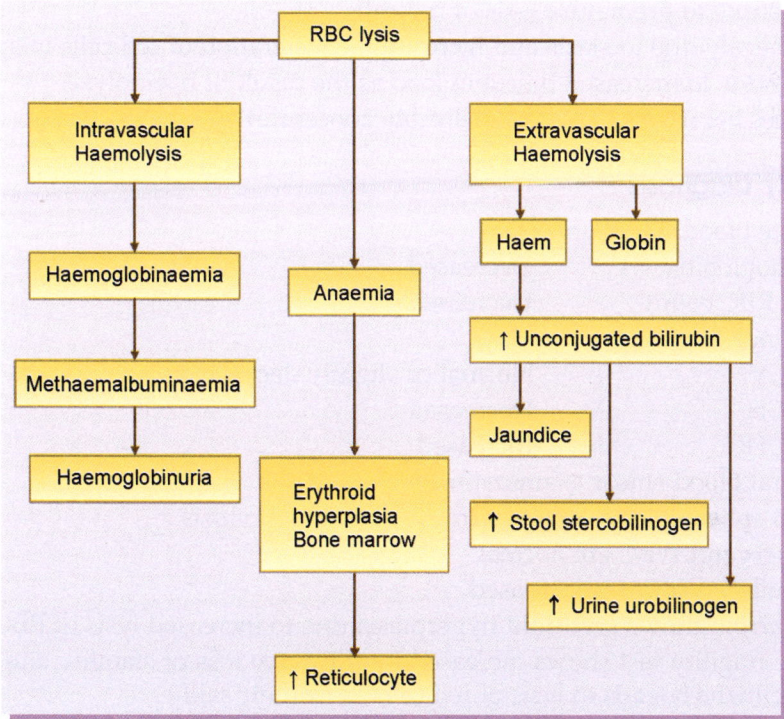

Fig. 15.5: Haemolytic anaemia

HEREDITARY SPHEROCYTOSIS

Inherited disease characterized by intrinsic defect in red cell membrane rendering spheroidal shape of red cell which is less deformable, as the result, they are more likely to be sequestrated and destroyed by spleen.

Molecular Pathology

- Spectrin, ankyrin, protein 4.1 and band 3 are cytoskeletal proteins responsible for the maintenance of normal shape, strength and flexibility of red cells.
- Deficiency of spectrin due to genetic defect results in loss of stability and flexibility of cell membrane.
- Red cell exposed to sheer stress in circulation leads to loss of membrane fragment result in spheroidal shape.
- Spheroidal red cells are sequestrated in narrow splenic cord, and subsequently red cells are destroyed.
- Extravascular haemolysis in spleen results in release of large amount of haemoglobin which is converted into bilirubin and carried to liver for conjugation and excreted in bile.

Clinical Features

- Anaemia due to premature lysis of red cells
- Splenomegaly due to stasis and increased sequestration of red cells in spleen
- Jaundice due to increased bilirubin load as the result of haemolysis
- Gallstones because of increased bilirubin concentration in bile

Laboratory Diagnosis

1. Complete blood cell count
   - Haemoglobin   Decreased
   - Total RBC count   Decreased
   - RBC indices

     MCV   Normal or slightly decreased

     MCH   Decreased

     MCHC   Increased
2. Peripheral blood smear examination reveals
   - Micro spherocytosis, hypochromasia, and anisocytosis
   - Platelets and WBC are normal
   - Reticulocyte count is increased
3. Bone marrow shows erythroid hyperplasia due to increased lysis of RBC.
4. Osmotic fragility test shows increased fragility due loss of stability and flexibility of red cell which leads to lysis of red cells in isotonic saline.
5. Direct Coombs' test is negative, since lysing antibodies are absent.
6. S. bilirubin is increased leading to jaundice.

SICKLE CELL DISEASE

It is hereditary haemoglobinopathy characterized by production of structurally abnormal haemoglobin (HbS) leading to haemolytic anaemia.

Pathology

A point mutation leading to substitution of glutamic acid by valine at 6th position in globin chain of haemoglobin molecule, results in abnormal haemoglobin known as haemoglobin S.

Pathophysiology (Fig. 15.6)

- Haemoglobin S (HbS) in deoxygenation states is aggregated and gets polymerized to form of haemoglobin fibers
- Haemoglobin fibers are precipitated over cell membrane resulting in detachment of membrane cytoskeleton and loss of water and potassium from cell
- Such dehydrated red cells assume sickle shape
- Free flowing haemoglobin in oxygenated state is converted into viscous gel on deoxygenation
- Sickle shape affects the flexibility and formability and exhibit increase adhesiveness Sickle cells therefore undergo extravascular haemolysis in spleen and cause vascular stasis leading to infarction of tissue.

Factors affecting the sickling are
- Amount of HbS—Heterozygous conditions (sickle cell trait) do not shows sickling except under severe hypoxia
- Interaction with other Hb—HbF inhibits polymerization, while HbD and HbC promote sickling
- pH—Fall in pH increases sickling
- Oxygen concentration—Decreased oxygen concentration increases sickling

Clinical Features

- Severe anaemia and generalized impairment of growth and development
- Vaso-occlusive complications causing ischaemic damage
- Chronic hyperbilirubinaemia
- Impaired splenic function and autosplenectomy due to hypoxic injury, stasis and congested red pulp
- Vaso-occlusive crisis
  - Aplastic crisis due to parvovirus infection
  - Splenic crisis due to sequestration of red cells in splenic cords

Laboratory Diagnosis

1. Complete blood cell count
   - Haemoglobin   Decreased
   - Total RBC count   Decreased

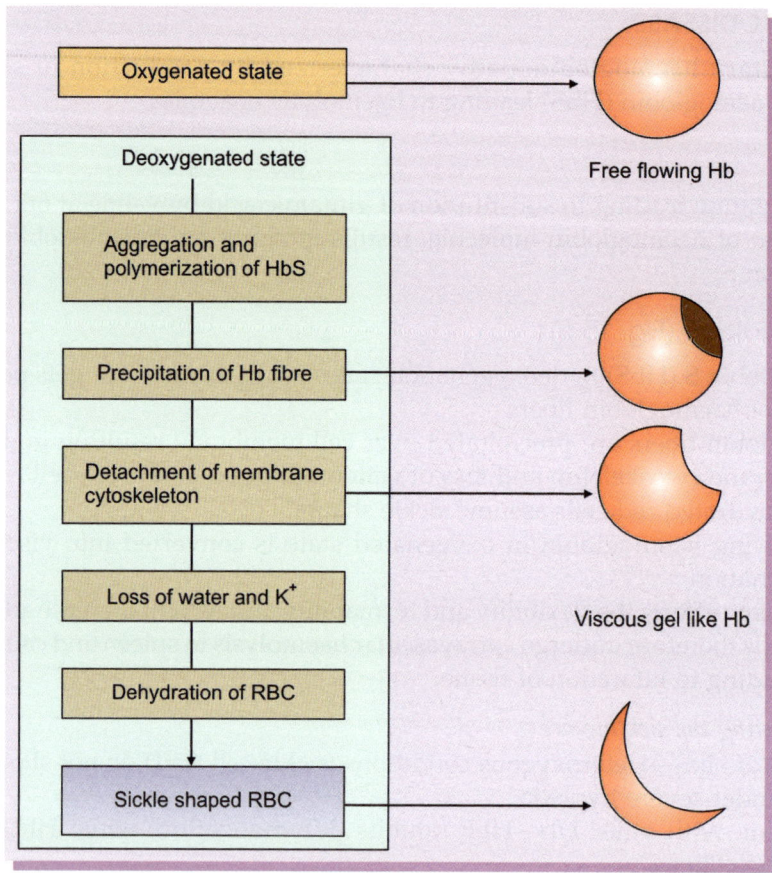

Fig. 15.6: Mechanism of sickling

RBC indices
- MCV   Normal or slightly decreased
- MCH   Decreased
- MCHC   Increased

2. Peripheral blood smear: PBF examination reveals presence of sickle cells, Howell-Jolly bodies, and nucleated RBCs. Platelets and WBC are normal. Reticulocyte count is increased.
3. Sickling test: It is based on principle that reducing substances like sodium metabisulfite which create deoxygenated state increases the sickling tendency.
4. Solubility test: Reducing substances like sodium dithionite give clear solution when mixed with HbA, while turbid solution with HbS.
5. Hb electrophoresis: Shows
   - Decreased or absent HbA
   - Increased HbS
   - Increased HbF (compensatory)
6. Osmotic fragility test: Reveal decreased fragility.

GLUCOSE 6 PHOSPHO DEHYDROGENASE DEFICIENCY (G6PD DEFICIENCY)

Role of G6DP (Fig. 15.7)

- Normally red cells are protected from oxidants by reduced glutathione which is generated by HMP shunt.
- In G6PD deficiency adequate reduced glutathione are not made available resulting in oxidation and precipitation of haemoglobin in the cell forming Heinz bodies.
- G6PD enzyme provides adequate NADPH for the reduction of glutathione.

Genetic Variants of G6PD

G6PD gene is located on X chromosome; therefore deficiency is sex linked affecting only males, female act as carrier and remains asymptomatic. More than 400 variants have been identified. Normal variant is type B. Black has normal variant type A+. Clinically significant variant is type A−. It offers protection against malaria.

Causes of Haemolysis

Drugs like antimalarial, sulfonamides, phenacetin, and aspirin. Infections like viral hepatitis, pneumonia, typhoid fever. Food material like Fava beans.

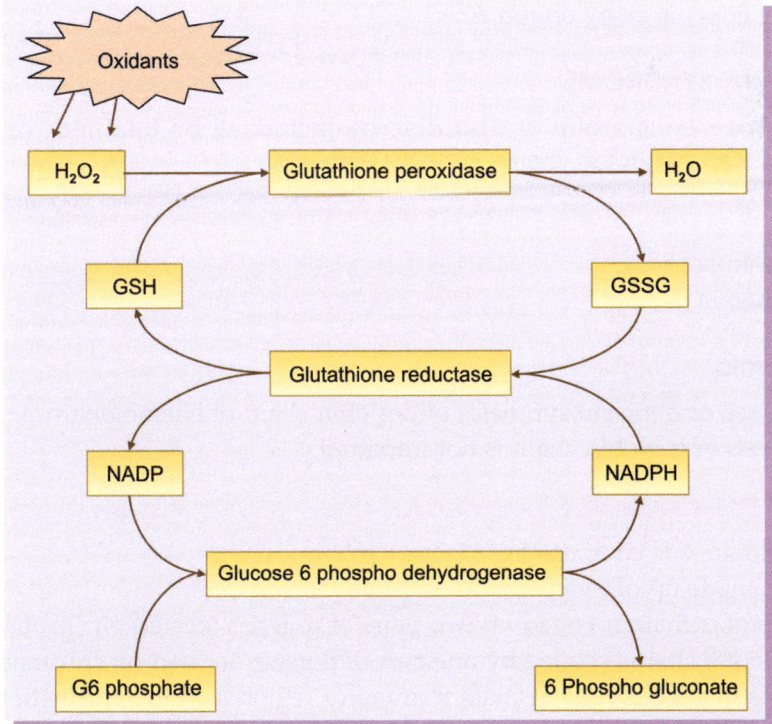

Fig. 15.7: Pathway of protection against oxidants and role of G6PD

Mechanism of Haemolysis

- Free radicals like H_2O_2 induce oxidation of sulfhydryl group of globin chain.
- Denatured Hb results in precipitation as Heinz bodies which cause deformity in red cells and undergo intravascular haemolysis.
- In spleen these Heinz bodies are plucked by macrophages leading to loss of membrane resulting in spheroidal shape which are liable to be destroyed by extravascular haemolysis.

Laboratory Diagnosis

During acute Haemolytic phase
- Rapid fall in haematocrit
- Haemoglobinaemia, haemoglobinuria and unconjugated hyperbilirubinaemia
- Heinz body demonstration in peripheral blood by supravital stains like crystal violet
- During recovery phase reticulocytes are increased

Between crisis phase
No anaemia, but red cell survival is reduced

G6PD assay by
- Indirect method like methemoglobin method
- Direct by enzyme assay on red cells

THALASSEMIA SYNDROME

It is a heterogeneous group of disorders characterized by total lack or decreased synthesis of α- or β- globin chain of haemoglobin A.

Types

1. α Thalassemia
2. β Thalassemia

β Thalassemia

- Total lack or deficient synthesis of β-globin chain of haemoglobin A
- Synthesis of α-globin chain is not impaired.

Molecular Pathology of α Thalassemia

- Haemoglobin A is composed of Haem + globin.
- Globin is made up of two α chains and two β chains
- Synthesis of α chain is coded by two pairs of α-genes located on chromosome 16.
- Synthesis of β chain is coded by one pair of β-genes located on chromosome 11.
- Mutations in genetic code at chain terminator region lead to nonfunctional β- gene labeled as β°
- Mutations in genetic code at promoter region leads to defective β-gene labeled as β⁺

Three types of β Thalassemia may be seen depending on genotype

Thalassemia major

- Homozygous β° Thalassemia   β°/β° genotype
- Homozygous β$^+$ Thalassemia   β$^+$/β$^+$ genotype
- Double heterozygous   β°/β$^+$ genotype

Thalassemia minor/trait

- Heterozygous   β°/β genotype or β$^+$/β genotype

Pathogenesis (Fig. 15.8)

- Impaired β-globin synthesis leads to anaemia by two mechanisms
- Lack or reduced haemoglobin A synthesis due to deficient β- globin chain
- Free unpaired α- chain get precipitated in normoblasts leading to apoptotic death of red cell precursors (ineffective erythropoiesis)
- Red cells which bear precipitated α- chain, if escape from bone marrow, then they are captured in spleen and phagocytosed (haemolysis)
- Anaemia stimulated erythropoiesis in bone marrow produce skeletal abnormalities
- Ineffective erythropoiesis cause excessive iron absorption coupled with massive blood transfusion leads to haemochromatosis

Clinical Features

β *Thalassemia Major*

- Most common type of β thalassemia is found in Mediterranean countries, part of Africa, India, and Southeast Asia
- Manifestations begin at 6–9 months after birth, when HbF starts decreasing
- Severe anaemia requires repeated blood transfusions, if not given, leads to growth retardation and early death
- Bossing of frontal bone and maxillary prominences due to extramedullary erythropoiesis create a peculiar thalassemic facies
- Hepatosplenomegaly is seen due to haemolysis and extra medullary erythropoiesis
- Recurrent infections, spontaneous fractures, leg ulcers may occur
- In repeatedly transfused patients secondary haemochromatosis is seen

β *Thalassemia Minor*

Usually asymptomatic, mild or no anaemia

Laboratory Diagnosis of β Thalassemia Major

1. Complete blood cell count
   - Haemoglobin   Very low 2–3 gm/dl
   - Total RBC count   Decreased

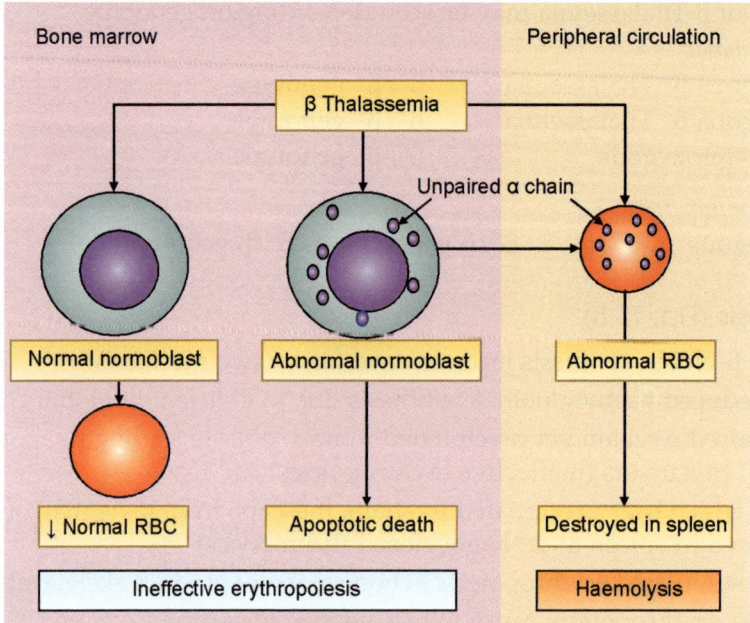

Fig. 15.8: Pathogenesis of β thalassemia

- RBC indices
MCV	Decreased
MCH	Decreased
MCHC	Decreased

  Platelets are normal or increased
  WBC is normal or increased
  Reticulocyte count increased

2. Peripheral blood smear examination reveals severe microcytosis, hypochromasia, marked aniso-poikilocytosis, basophilic stippling, teardrop cell, target cells, fragmented red cells. Numerous nucleated RBCs are seen.
3. Bone marrow shows normoblastic erythroid hyperplasia, with ineffective erythropoiesis. Increased iron in reticuloendothelial cell with siderotic granules in normoblasts.
4. Haemoglobin electrophoresis
   - HbA —markedly diminished or absent
   - HbA$_2$—normal or diminished or increased
   - HbF—markedly increased
5. Biochemical tests
   - S. unconjugated bilirubin high
   - Urinary urobilinogen increased
   - S. transferrin saturation high
   - Ferritin high
6. Osmotic fragility test shows decreased osmotic fragility of red cells.

Laboratory Diagnosis of β Thalassemia Minor/Trait

1. Complete blood cell count
   - Haemoglobin slightly low
   - Total RBC count normal
   - RBC indices

MCV	Decreased
MCH	Decreased
MCHC	Decreased

     Platelets are normal or increased

     WBC is normal or increased

     Reticulocyte count increased
2. Peripheral blood smear examination reveals

   Mild microcytosis, hypochromasia, mild aniso-poikilocytosis

   Basophilic stippling, teardrop cell, target cells, fragmented red cells are present but less prominent. Numerous nucleated RBCs are less frequent.
3. Bone marrow shows mild normoblastic erythroid hyperplasia.
4. Haemoglobin electrophoresis
   - HbA—slightly diminished
   - HbA$_2$—normal or increased
   - HbF—normal or slightly increased
5. Osmotic fragility test shows decreased osmotic fragility of red cells.

α Thalassemia

- Total lack or deficient synthesis of α- globin chain of haemoglobin A
- Synthesis of β-globin chain is not impaired

Molecular Pathology of α Thalassemia

- Haemoglobin A is composed of haem + globin.
- Globin is made up of two α- chains and two β- chains
- Synthesis of α- chain is coded by two pairs of α-genes located on chromosome 16.
- Synthesis of β- chain is coded by one pair of β-genes located on chromosome 11.
- Deletion of α-gene is responsible for α thalassemia.

Four types of α thalassemia may be seen depending on genotype

α Thalassemia	Genotype
1. Hydrops foetalis	- -/- -
2. HbH disease	- -/- α
3. ? Thalassemia trait	- -/α α (Asian)
	- α/- α (black African)
4. Silent carrier	- α/α α

Pathogenesis

- Impaired α-globin synthesis leads to anaemia by two mechanisms
- Lack or reduced haemoglobin A synthesis due to deficient α-globin chain
- Free unpaired non-α chain get precipitated in normoblasts leading to apoptotic death of red cell precursors (ineffective erythropoiesis)
- Red cells which bear precipitated non-α chain, if escape from bone marrow, then they are captured in spleen and phagocytosed (haemolysis)
- In newborn excess of γ- chain form tetramer $γ_4$ called Bart haemoglobin
- In adult tetramer of β- chain are formed called haemoglobin H
- Non-α chains in general form more soluble and less toxic aggregates, the haemolytic anaemia tend to be less severe than β thalassemia

Clinical Features

1. Hydrops Foetalis

- Haemoglobin Bart formed by excess of γ- chains have high oxygen affinity but is unstable and lead to intrauterine death of foetus.
- Fetus appears pale, generalized edema with massive hepatosplenomegaly.

2. Haemoglobin H Disease

- It is mainly seen in Asian population and rarely in African.
- Haemoglobin H has high affinity for oxygen but not stable, therefore patient have moderately severe anaemia.
- Other symptoms of thalassemia in general are seen.

3. α Thalassemia Trait

- Asian and African type shows similar clinical features of minimal or no anaemia.
- Offspring of African heterozygous genotype mating will not result in HbH disease or hydrops foetalis, while Asian type will result in severe form of α thalassemia.

4. Silent Carrier

These patients are normal and asymptomatic.

Laboratory Diagnosis of α Thalassemia Major

1. Complete blood cell count
    - Haemoglobin   Low
    - Total RBC count   Decreased
    - RBC indices
        MCV   Decreased
        MCH   Decreased
        MCHC   Decreased

Platelets are normal or increased

WBC is normal or increased

Reticulocyte count is increased

2. Peripheral blood smear examination reveals microcytosis, hypochromasia, moderate aniso-poikilocytosis, basophilic stippling, teardrop cell, target cells, fragmented red cells. Numerous nucleated RBCs are seen.

3. Bone marrow shows normoblastic erythroid hyperplasia, with ineffective erythropoiesis.

4. Haemoglobin electrophoresis
   - HbA—Markedly diminished or absent
   - HbH—Abnormal haemoglobin in adult
   - Hb Bart—Abnormal haemoglobin in foetus

5. Biochemical tests
   - S. unconjugated bilirubin high
   - Urinary urobilinogen increased

6. Osmotic fragility test shows decreased osmotic fragility of red cells.

16

Haemorrhagic Diseases

DEFINITION

- **Bleeding disorder**—Bleeding due to capillary or platelet defect is known as bleeding disorder.
- **Coagulation disorder**—Haemorrhagic diathesis due to defect in mechanism of coagulation is known as coagulation disorder.
- **Haemorrhage**—It is extravasation of blood because of rupture of blood vessel.
- **Haematoma**—Blood enclosed within a tissue space due to haemorrhage is called haematoma.
- **Petechial haemorrhage**—Bleeding points over skin, mucous membrane and serosa measuring 1–2 mm because of increased intravascular pressure, decreased platelet counts or defect in platelet function is known as petechial haemorrhage.
- **Purpura**—Larger haemorrhagic patches measuring >3 mm in size, because of vasculitis or increased vascular fragility is called purpura.
- **Ecchymoses**—Subcutaneous haematoma measuring >1–2 cm in size is called ecchymoses. There is color change from red to yellow to brown with time.
- **Haemothorax, haemoperitoneum, haem arthrosis**—These are terms used for accumulation of blood in body cavities like pleura/peritoneal cavity/joint.

Mechanism of Haemostasis

Haemostasis involve three components
1. Vascular component
2. Platelet component
3. Coagulation component

Primary Haemostasis

- Vascular component
- Platelet component

Secondary Haemostasis

Coagulation component.

1. *Role of Vascular Component*

Procoagulant Function

- vWF synthesized by endothelium binds platelet to collagen
- Tissue factor secreted by endothelium activate clotting factors
- Endothelium secretes inhibitors of plasminogen activators

Anticoagulant Function

- Anti platelet effect induced by endothelial PGI (prostacyclin), nitric oxide and ADP
- Anticoagulant effect induced by heparin like molecules and thrombomodulin. Fibrinolytic effect by tissue plasminogen activator.

2. *Role of Platelet Component*

Seventy percent of platelets remain in circulation while 30% in spleen.

Adhesion of platelet to endothelium is facilitated by

- von Willebrand factor synthesized and released by endothelium
- Subendothelial collagen tissue
- ADP and thromboxane A_2

Aggregation of platelet is facilitated by thromboxane A_2 synthesized from arachidonic acid by cyclooxygenase and thromboxan synthetase. Adhesion and aggregation of platelet results in formation of primary haemostatic plug which seals off the vascular breach and arrest bleeding.

3. *Role of Coagulation Component*

Coagulation cascade may be divided into three pathways:

1. Intrinsic pathway, screened by activated partial thromboplastin time (aPTT) estimation
2. Extrinsic pathway, screened by prothrombin time (PT)
3. Common pathway defect in any of the three components may lead to bleeding disorder

BLEEDING DISORDERS

A. Due to Vessel Wall Abnormality

Haemorrhage occurs due to defect/damage in blood vessels. Platelet number, function of platelet and coagulation system all appear normal.

Causes

- Infections like meningococcemia, septicemia, and endocarditis
- Drugs which cause vasculitis due to hypersensitivity reaction
- Systemic hypersensitivity reaction (Henoch-Schönlein purpura)
- Amyloid infiltrate in blood vessel

- Deficiency of vitamin C (scurvy)
- Hereditary haemorrhagic telangiectasia

Clinical Features

- Petechial haemorrhage, purpura over skin and mucus membrane
- Haemorrhage in muscle, bone and joints
- Menorrhagia, epistaxis, haematuria, haematemesis and melena

Laboratory diagnosis

- Platelet count (PC)   Normal
- Bleeding time (BT)   Normal
- Clotting time (CT)   Normal
- Prothrombin time (PT)   Normal
- Activated partial thromboplastin time (aPTT)   Normal

B. Due to Platelet Abnormality

Thrombocytopenia

Haemorrhage occurs because of decreased number of platelets in circulation is known as thrombocytopenia. Thrombocytopenia is due to known reasons.

Normal platelet count— 1.5 to 4.5 lac per cumm

Causes of Thrombocytopenia

1. Impaired production (bone marrow diseases)
2. Decreased survival (destruction of platelets)
   - By antiplatelet antibodies
   - Drug induced
   - HIV associated
   - By mechanical injury
3. Sequestration in spleen (hypersplenism)
4. Dilutional (massive stored blood transfusion)

Laboratory Diagnosis

- Platelet count (PC)   Decreased (normal 1.5–4.0 lac/cumm)
- Bleeding time (BT)   Increased
- Clotting time (CT)   Normal
- Prothrombin time (PT)   Normal
- Activated partial   Normal
  thromboplastin time (aPTT)

Clinical Features

- Small petechial haemorrhage or large ecchymotic patches are seen over skin and/or mucus membrane.

- Bleeding into nervous system constitute major hazard
- Epistaxis, bleeding gums, hematemesis, haemoptysis, and haematuria are other manifestations

IDIOPATHIC THROMBOCYTOPAENIC PURPURA (ITP)

Thrombocytopaenia with the absence of known causes is known as idiopathic thrombocytopenia. It is supposed to be due to immune mediated destruction of platelet therefore also known as primary immune thrombocytopaenic purpura or autoimmune thrombocytopenic purpura. It is of two types depending upon the age group involved and onset of the disease.

Types

1. Acute idiopathic thrombocytopaenic purpura
2. Chronic idiopathic thrombocytopaenic purpura

Features	Acute Idiopathic thrombo-cytopaenic purpura	Chronic Idiopathic thrombocytopaenic purpura
Age	Children, 2–6 years	Adult 20–40 years
Sex	None	Female: Male ratio 3:1
Prior infection	Common	Uncommon
Onset of bleeding	Abrupt	Insidious
Platelet count	Less than 20000/cumm	30000–80000/cumm
Eosinophilia and lymphocytosis	Common	Uncommon
Duration of disease	2–6 weeks	Months to years
Spontaneous remission	Occurs in majority cases, 20% progress to chronic ITP	Uncommon

Pathogenesis

- Autoantibodies (IgG type) are formed against platelet membrane glycoprotein, which bind to circulating platelets.
- Opsonised platelets are recognized through Fc portion of antibodies by macrophages and phagocytosed.
- Phagocytosis occurs in spleen leading to splenomegaly, therefore splenectomy improves the condition.

Laboratory Diagnosis

- CBC shows normocytic, normochromic anaemia due to bleeding
- Platelet count is reduced, with the appearance of large platelets in the circulation
- Platelet count (PC)   Decreased (normal 1.5–4.0 lac/cumm)
- Bleeding time (BT)   Increased
- Clotting time (CT)   Normal
- Prothrombin time (PT)   Normal

- Activated partial thromboplastin time (aPTT) normal
- Antiplatelet antibodies are detected
- Bone marrow shows increased number of megakaryocytes and its precursors

COAGULATION DISORDERS

Coagulation disorders occur due to defect in coagulation mechanism. It may be genetic or acquired.

A. Hereditary

1. X-Linked Recessive Traits

- Haemophilia A
- Haemophilia B

2. Autosomal Recessive Traits

- Factor XI deficiency
- Prothrombin deficiency
- Factor V, VII, X, XII, XIII deficiency
- Afibrinogenemia/hypofibrinogenemia

3. Autosomal Dominant Traits

- von Willebrand's disease
- Dysfibrinogenemia
- Passovoy factor deficiency

4. Combined

- Associated with haemophilia
- Involving vitamin K dependent factors

5. Miscellaneous

- Prekallikrein deficiency
- HMW kininogen deficiency

B. Acquired

1. Deficiency of Vitamin K Dependent Factors

- Haemorrhagic disease of newborn
- Biliary obstruction
- Malabsorption of vitamin K
- Nutritional deficiency
- Drugs like coumarins, broad spectrum antibiotics, and cholestyramine

2. Accelerated Destruction of Coagulation Factors

- Disseminated intravascular coagulation (DIC)
- Fibrinolysis in liver disease, thrombotic agents, tumors, post surgery

3. Inhibitors of Coagulation

- Specific inhibitor
- Lupus anticoagulants
- Antithrombin
- Paraproteinaemias

4. Miscellaneous

- After massive transfusion
- Antibiotic, antineoplastic agents
- Congenital heart diseases, amyloidosis, nephritic syndrome, leukaemia

HAEMOPHILIA

It is a hereditary disease affecting male children with serious bleeding tendencies due to deficiency of factor VIII (Anti-haemophilic factor).

Pathophysiology (Fig. 16.1)

- In circulation factor VIII is bound to von Willebrand factor (vWF)
- Seven different mutations in haemophilia gene present over X chromosome leads to decreased amount or decreased activity of factor VIII
- Functional unit of factor VIII is VIIIC
- Incidence is 1 in 20000

Clinical Features

- Massive haemorrhage after trivial injury and easy bruising is seen commonly
- Spontaneous bleeding in joints (haemarthrosis) is a debilitating manifestation. Haemorrhage with organized inflammation leads to chronic haemophilic arthropathy
- Subcutaneous, intramuscular retroperitoneal haematoma leads to spasm, pain and limitation of mobility
- Gastrointestinal and genitourinary bleeding is quite common
- Splenomegaly is seen in 40% patients

Laboratory Diagnosis

1. Complete Blood Count Shows Normocytic, Normochromic Anaemia due to Bleeding

Platelet count is normal, megakaryocytes are normal or increased.

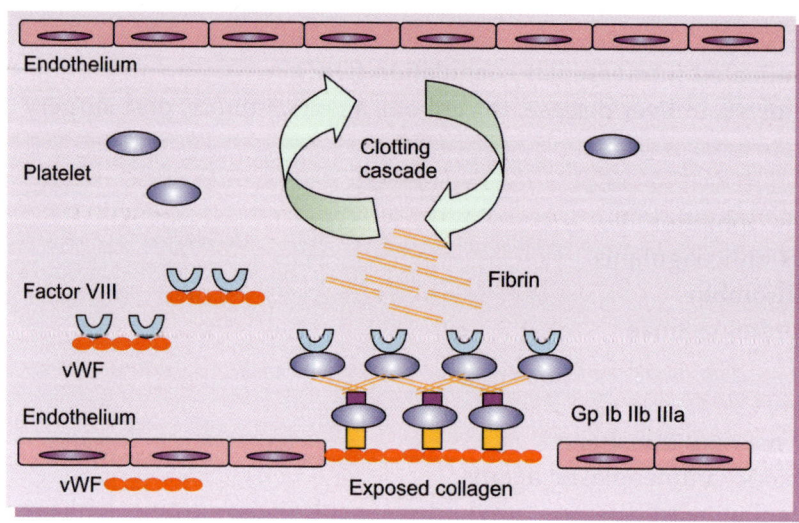

Fig. 16.1: Interaction vWF and factor VIII in haemostasis

2. Coagulation Profile

Bleeding time (BT)	Normal
Clotting time (CT)	Prolonged
Prothrombin time (PT)	Normal

Activated partial thromboplastin time (aPTT) is prolonged

3. Factor VIII Assay

Severe deficiency	<2 U/dl
Moderate deficiency	2–5 U/dl
Mild deficiency	>5 U/dl

Detection of carrier

Detection of subnormal level of factor VIIIC

Ratio of VIIIC to vWF 0.18–0.9 (Normal: 0.74–2.2)

Haemophilia in female is seen in heterozygous carrier when X chromosome is inactivated or new mutant gene appears in carrier. Female children of carrier female and affected male may lead to manifestations of haemophilia.

VON WILLEBRAND'S DISEASE

It is hereditary autosomal dominant bleeding and clotting compound disorder due to deficiency of von Willebrand factor. Decreased vWF is associated with decreased factor VIII in blood; hence defect in platelet function and coagulation pathway both are present.

Pathophysiology

- vWF is synthesized by endothelial cells and megakaryocytes
- vWF facilitates platelet adhesion, act as carrier of factor VIII and also stabilizes factor VIII
- vWF is of three types I, II, and III. Type IIC and type III are autosomal recessive, rest are autosomal dominant. Gene encoding for vWF is present on chromosome 12

Clinical Features

Spontaneous mild to massive bleeding, easy bruising, epistaxis, menorrhagia, bleeding following minor procedures are seen.

Laboratory Diagnosis

- Platelet count (PC)   Normal
- Bleeding time (BT)   Increased
- Clotting time (CT)   Increased
- Prothrombin time (PT)   Normal
- Activated partial thromboplastin time (aPTT) prolonged
- vWF assay shows decreased level
- Factor VIIIC level is decreased
- Ristocetin induced platelet aggregation, which is dependent on vWF, is abnormal

17

Leukaemia

Definition

Leukaemia is malignant transformation of blood forming cells in bone marrow and lymphoid tissue. Leukaemic cells spread in peripheral blood and infiltrates various organs.

Classification (FAB–French–American–British)

1. Acute leukaemia
   A. Myeloid cells
   B. Lymphoid cells
2. Chronic leukaemia
   A. Myeloid cells
   B. Lymphoid cells

ACUTE LEUKAEMIA

Acute leukaemia is characterized by accumulation of immature lymphoid/myeloid cells in bone marrow, lymphoid tissue and other organs.

Etiological Factors

1. Familial and genetic
   - Down syndrome
   - Ataxia telangiectasia
2. Drugs and toxins
   - Cytotoxic drugs like alkylating agents
   - Benzene
3. Retrovirus
   - Human T cell leukaemia-lymphoma virus (HTLV)
4. Ionizing radiations
   - α- β- γ- radiation, X-rays

5. Immunological
   Immune deficiency states

Grading and Nomenclature of Acute Leukaemia
(French-American-British classification)

Grading	Acute myeloid leukaemia
M0	Minimally differentiated
M1	Myeloblastic leukaemia without maturation
M2	Myeloblastic leukaemia with maturation
M3	Hypergranular promyelocytic leukaemia
M4	Myelomonocytic leukaemia
M4Eo	Variant, increased eosinophils in marrow
M5	Monocytic leukaemia
M6	Erythroleukaemia
M7	Megakaryoblastic leukaemia
Grading	Acute lymphoid leukaemia
L1	Small lymphoblastic, homogeneous population
L2	Small and large lymphoblastic, heterogeneous population
L3 (Burkitt's)	Large lymphoblastic homogeneous population

Differences between Acute Myeloid and Acute Lymphoid Leukaemia

Features	Ac. lymphoid leukaemia	Acute myeloid leukaemia
1. Age group involved	Children	Young adults
2. Lymphadenopathy	Prominent	Less common
3. Hepatosplenomegaly	Common	Less common
4. CNS, testis, eye infiltration	More common	Less common
5. Bleeding tendency	Less common	More common
6. Gum involvement	Not seen	Gum hypertrophy (M5)
7. Leukaemic blast cells	Lymphoblasts	Myeloblasts
8. TdT (terminal deoxy-nucleotidyl transferase)	Often positive	Negative

Clinical Features of Acute Leukaemia

1. Symptoms due to marrow failure
   - Anaemia
   - Bleeding manifestations
   - Infections
   - Fever
2. Symptoms due to organ infiltration
   - Bone pain and sternal tenderness
   - Lymphadenopathy

- Hepatomegaly
- Splenomegaly
- Leukaemic infiltrate in meninges, brain, kidney, gums, skin

Laboratory Diagnosis

1. Complete Blood Counts

Haemoglobin	Decreased
Total RBC count	Normal or reduced

RBC indices

MCV	Normal
MCH	Normal or reduced
MCHC	Normal or reduced
Reticulocyte count	Increased

Total leukocyte count may be normal or markedly raised. Peripheral blood smear shows numerous blast cells (lymphoid or myeloid). Platelet count is markedly decreased (Fig. 17.1).

2. Bone Marrow

Bone marrow is hypercellular and normal elements are replaced by leukaemic blast cells. Erythropoietic cells and megakaryocytes are reduced in number. Presence of more than 20% of blast cell is diagnostic of acute leukaemia. Predominant cell type determines the lymphoid or myeloid type leukaemia.

3. Lymph Nodes

Lymph nodes are infiltrated by blast leukaemic cells. Lymph nodes are predominantly involved in acute lymphocytic leukaemia.

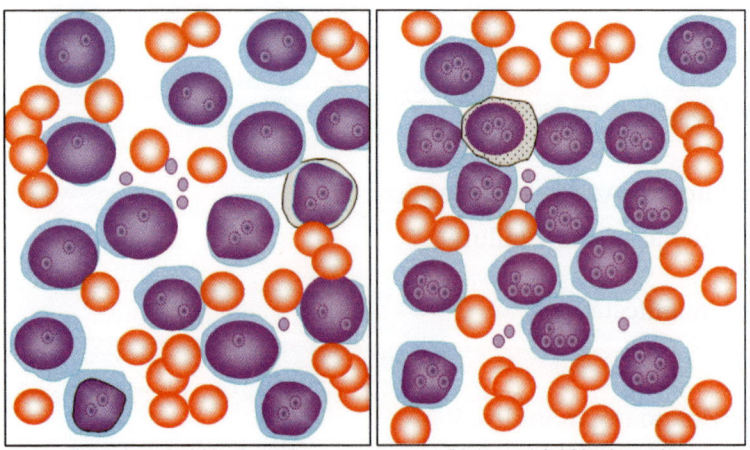

Acute lymphoid leukaemia   Acute myeloid leukaemia

Fig. 17.1: Acute leukaemia

4. Other Organs

Liver, kidneys spleen and all organs get infiltrated by leukaemic cells.

CHRONIC LEUKAEMIA

It is characterized by neoplastic proliferation of myeloid/lymphoid cell with mature cell in peripheral blood, bone marrow, lymphoid tissue and other organs.

Classification (FAB–French-American-British)

A. Chronic myelocytic leukaemia
  • Philadelphia positive
  • Philadelphia negative, break point cluster positive (BCR+)
  • Philadelphia negative, break point cluster negative (BCR-)
  • Eosinophilic leukaemia
B. Chronic lymphocytic leukaemia
  • Common B cell
  • Rare T cell
  • Hairy cell
  • Prolymphocytic

CHRONIC MYELOID LEUKAEMIA (CML)

Chronic myeloid leukaemia is a myeloproliferative disease characterized by excessive proliferation of myeloid cells. **Natural course of disease** may be divided into three phases
1. Chronic stable phase
2. Accelerated phase
3. Blast crisis phase

1. Chronic Stable Phase

Age incidence–middle age (30–60 years)

Symptoms

A. **In initial stage** patient remain asymptomatic.
B. **Later on** symptoms develop
  1. *Symptoms due to massive splenomegaly:* Abdominal distension, dyspepsia, reflux esophagitis, dysphonia, dragging sensation in left hypochondrium, hepatomegaly often accompanies the splenomegaly.
  2. *Symptoms due to hypermetabolic state:* Fever, weight loss, night sweat, heat intolerance.
  3. Symptoms due to anaemia: Fatigability, weakness, anorexia.
C. **Lately** bleeding manifestations

Laboratory Diagnosis

1. Complete blood counts

Haemoglobin	Decreased
Total RBC count	Normal or reduced
RBC indices	
MCV	Normal
MCH	Normal or reduced
MCHC	Normal or reduced
Reticulocyte count	Increased
Total leukocyte count	is markedly raised

2. Peripheral blood smear: Shows granulocytic precursor cells predominantly myelocyte and metamyelocyte. Myeloblasts are less than 10%. Basophilia and eosinophilia may be seen. Platelet count is normal or reduced (Fig. 17.2).

3. Bone marrow examination: Hypercellular with marked proliferation of granulocytic cells.

4. Philadelphia chromosome: It is reciprocal translocation of long arm of chromosome 9 and chromosome 22. It is positive in majority of cases of CML (Fig. 17.3).

5. Leukocytic alkaline phosphatase is very low (c.f. leukocytosis where it is very high)

2. Accelerated Phase of CML

It is characterized by significant anaemia, increased spleen, increased total leukocyte count and more precursor cells, basophilia.

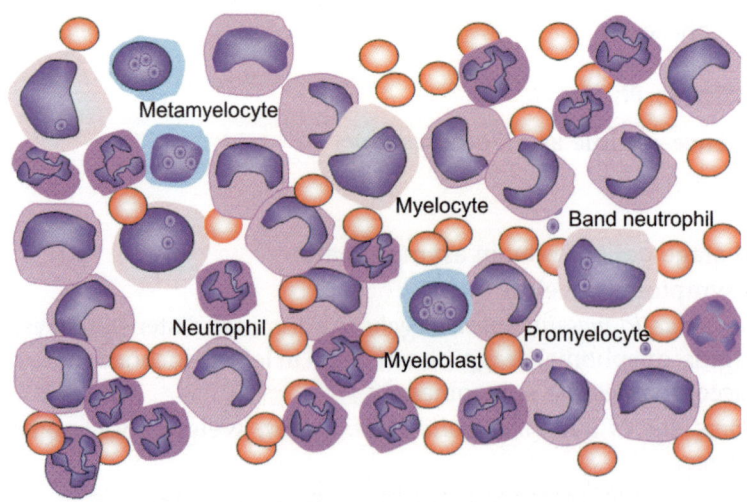

Fig. 17.2: Chronic myeloid leukaemia

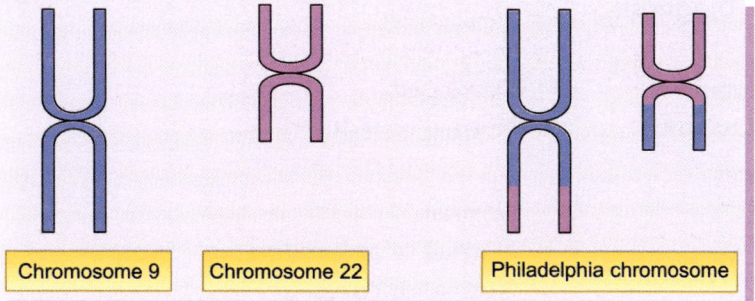

Fig. 17.3: Philadelphia chromosome

3. Blast Crisis Phase of CML

Blast crisis phase is transformation of chronic leukaemia into acute leukaemia. CML may transform to blast crisis through accelerated phase or directly without accelerated phase. CML may transform into:

- Acute myeloid leukaemia called **myeloid blast crisis**
- Acute lymphoblastic leukaemia called **lymphoid blast crisis**

Blast crisis is characterized by:
- Sudden increase in spleen size
- Generalized lymphadenopathy
- Anaemia and bleeding tendencies with the appearance of numerous blast cells in peripheral blood
- Disease does not respond to treatment

CHRONIC LYMPHOCYTIC LEUKAEMIA (CLL)

Chronic lymphocytic leukaemia is characterized by persistent lymphocytosis (more than 1 lac/cumm) with infiltration in bone marrow spleen and bone marrow.

Types
- 95% cases are B cell chronic lymphocytic leukaemia
- 5% cases are T cell chronic lymphocytic leukaemia

Clinical Features
- Commonly seen after 50 years of age, predominantly in males
- Patient may be asymptomatic
- Generalized lymphadenopathy and hepatosplenomegaly
- Recurrent infections due to decreased amount of antibodies

Laboratory Diagnosis

1. Complete blood counts

Haemoglobin	Decreased
Total RBC count	Normal or reduced

RBC indices

MCV	Normal
MCH	Normal or reduced
MCHC	Normal or reduced
Reticulocyte count	Normal of Increased

Total leukocyte count is markedly raised (50000–200000/cumm)

2. Peripheral blood smear (Fig. 17.4)

Shows predominantly mature lymphocytes (>95%)

Platelet count is normal or reduced

3. Bone marrow examination

Hypercellular with infiltration of mature lymphocytes

Erythroid and myeloid precursors are decreased in number

4. Direct Coombs' test may be positive in 20% cases

Clinical Staging

Stage A	No anaemia or thrombocytopaenia
	Less than 3 areas of lymphoid involvement
Stage B	No anaemia or thrombocytopaenia
	More than 3 areas of lymphoid involvement
Stage C	Anaemia and/or thrombocytopaenia
	Less than 3 areas of lymphoid involvement

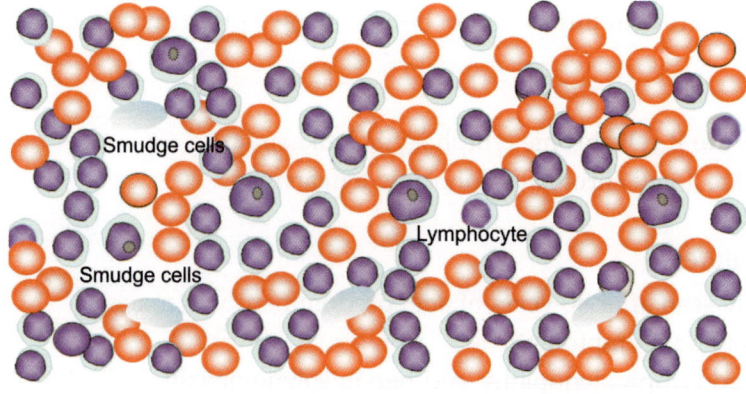

Fig. 17.4: Chronic lymphocytic leukaemia

MYELOPROLIFERATIVE DISORDERS

It is characterized by proliferation of multipotent haematopoietic stem cells, leading to following diseases
1. Chronic myeloid leukaemia (*already completed*)
2. Polycythemia vera
3. Myelofibrosis (agnogenic myeloid metaplasia)
4. Thrombocytosis

2. Polycythemia Vera

It is characterized by pancytosis, i.e. increased number of all three blood cells.

Classification

1. **Primary polycythemia vera** characterized by
   • Pancytosis with splenomegaly
   • Leukocytosis
   • Thrombocytosis
   • Decreased erythropoietin
2. **Secondary polycythemia vera** characterized by
   • Increased erythropoietin
     – Occurs at high altitude
     – Due to pulmonary disease
     – Due to smoking

Clinical Features

• Commonly seen in late middle ages
• Males are more affected than females
• It has a chronic course

Symptoms

a. **Hyperviscosity**—results in increased tendency of thrombosis
b. **Hypervolemia**—leads to increased risk of haemorrhage
c. **Hypermetabolism**—cause increased risk of calculus and gout
d. **Decreased cerebral perfusion**—cause headache, vertigo and visual disturbances
e. Splenomegaly

Laboratory Diagnosis

1. Complete blood counts
   • Haemoglobin—Increased >17.5 g% (M), >15.5 g% (F)
   • Total RBC count—Increased >6 million/cumm (M), >5.5 million/cumm (F)
   • Packed cell volume—Increased >55% (M), >47% (F)

- Reticulocyte count—Increased
- Total leukocyte count is raised (15000–25000/cumm)
- Platelet count increased with defective platelet function

2. Bone marrow shows panhyperplasia.

3. Myelofibrosis (Agnogenic Myeloid Metaplasia)

It is characterized by proliferation of haematopoietic neoplastic cells at multiple extramedullary sites with fibrosis in bone marrow.

Etiological Classification

A. Primary (idiopathic)
B. Secondary (marrow disorder due to chemicals and irradiation)

Clinical Features

It is commonly seen between the age of 40 and 70. Manifestations are

- Anaemia
- Hepatosplenomegaly
- Bleeding tendencies
- Lymphadenopathy

Laboratory Diagnosis

1. Complete blood counts
   - Haemoglobin—Ddecreased
   - Total RBC count—Decreased
   - Reticulocyte count—Increased
   - Total leukocyte count—Decreased or increased, with myeloid precursors in abundance, Blast cells are less than 10%
   - Platelet count—Increased (early phase) decreased (later on)
2. Peripheral blood smear
   - It shows aniso-poikilocytosis with oval and teardrop red cells, polychromasia and basophilic stippling
3. Bone marrow
   Early phase: Hypercellular with increase in all three cell lines, fibrosis is minimal.
   Late phase: Hypocellular with reduction in all three cell lines and marked fibrosis.
4. Extramedullary erythropoiesis
   Seen in liver and spleen, at times in lymph nodes, kidneys and adrenals
5. Leukocytic alkaline phosphatase—Elevated
6. Philadelphia chromosomes—Negative

4. Thrombocytosis

It is characterized by neoplastic proliferation of platelets

Clinical Features

- Arterial/venous thrombosis
- Easy bruisability following minor trauma
- Spontaneous bleeding
- Transient ischaemic attacks (TIA)

Laboratory Diagnosis

1. Complete blood counts
   - Haemoglobin—Normal or reduced
   - Total RBC count—Decreased
   - Reticulocyte count—Increased
   - Total leukocyte count—Normal
   - Platelet count increased, large platelets and megakaryocytes are seen
2. Bone marrow
   Large numbers of hyperdiploid megakaryocytes are seen with increased fibrosis.

18

Diseases of Lymph Node

Proliferative diseases of lymph nodes include
1. Reactive proliferation
2. Neoplastic proliferation

1. Reactive Lymphadenitis

Infectious and noninfectious inflammatory stimuli can cause reactive lymphadenitis.

A. Acute Nonspecific Lymphadenitis

It may be confined to local group of lymph node draining a focal infection or may be generalized due to systemic bacterial/viral infections.

Gross Features

Lymph nodes become tender and fluctuant, if abscess is formed. It may lead to sinus formation, if overlying skin is involved.

Microscopic Features

Large germinal centers are seen. Neutrophilic exudates may be seen in pyogenic infections. In severe cases follicles undergo necrosis resulting in formation of suppurative focus, i.e. abscess.

B. Chronic Nonspecific Lymphadenitis

Depending on causative agents three different patterns can be seen.

i. Follicular Hyperplasia

- It is associated with infections and inflammations which activate B lymphocyte.
- Lymphoid follicles are enlarged with prominent germinal centers, revealing scattered macrophages with tingible bodies and follicular dendritic cells.

ii. *Paracortical Hyperplasia*
- It is seen in viral infection, following vaccination and in drug reactions.
- Reactive changes are seen in paracortical T cell region.

iii. *Sinus Histiocytosis*
- Dilated lymphatic channels are seen lined by hypertrophied lining endothelium with increased number of macrophages.
- It is often seen in lymph nodes draining cancers.

2. Neoplastic Disease
- Neoplastic proliferation and infiltration of tumor cells in lymphoid tissue is known as lymphoma.
- Neoplastic proliferation and infiltration of lymphoid tumor cells in blood is known as lymphoid leukaemia (lymphosarcoma).

LYMPHOMA

It is characterized by neoplastic proliferation of lymphoid tissue. It is classified into two types:
- Hodgkin's lymphoma
- Non-Hodgkin's lymphoma

Hodgkin's Lymphoma

Hodgkin's lymphoma is characterized by neoplastic proliferation of lymphoid tissue accompanied with characteristic Reed-Sternberg cells.

Characteristic Features

It shows bimodal age distribution
- In young adults (15–35 years) and older adults (45–75 years)
- Presence of Reed-Sternberg cell is a diagnostic hallmark feature.

Reed-Sternberg Cell (RS cell)

It is a large (15–45 mm) cell with abundant cytoplasm and bilobed mirror image nucleus with prominent nucleoli. Sometimes multilobulation and multinucleation is seen called RS cell variants.

Reed-Sternberg Cell Variants (Fig. 18.1)

1. Mononuclear variant shows a single round to oblong nucleus with large nucleoli.
2. Lacunar cell shows delicate multilobated/folded nucleus with abundant pale clear cytoplasm, seen as halo around nucleus.
3. L and H variants.

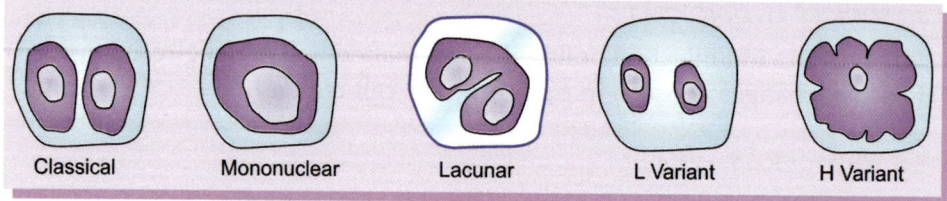

Fig. 18.1: RS cell variants

- Mummified Reed-Sternberg cell with pyknotic nucleus
- Popcorn like polypoid nucleus and inconspicuous nucleoli

Classification of Hodgkin's Lymphoma

1. Nodular Sclerosis (NS)
2. Mixed Cellularity (MC)
3. Lymphocytic Rich (LR)
4. Lymphocytic Depleted (LD)
5. Lymphocytic Predominant (LP)

   All types, except lymphocytic predominant type shows RS cells of same phenotype, lymphocytic predominant type shows B cell phenotype.

Etiopathogenesis

- Reed-Sternberg cell are thought to be of germinal center origin (B lymphocyte), rarely they arise from transformed T lymphocyte.
- In Reed-Sternberg cell episomes of Epstein-Barr virus are seen and such cells express latent membrane protein (LMP-1). LMP-1 protein has transformation activity by up-regulating NF-KB factor. NF-KB factor is responsible for activation of lymphocytes.
- NF-KB activation makes the cell to escape from apoptosis, hence, transformed cell persist as Reed-Sternberg cell. Reed-Sternberg cell release cytokines which leads to accumulation of reactive cell in the vicinity.

Gross Features

Rubbery, discrete, non tender, firm lymph nodes, on cutting appear homogeneous.

Microscopic Features

1. Nodular Sclerosis

- Lymph node is divided by fibrous septa in cellular sheets and lobules composed of lymphocytes, macrophages, and plasma cells.
- Peculiar Lacunar cells are seen frequently. Classical Reed-Sternberg cell are occasionally present.

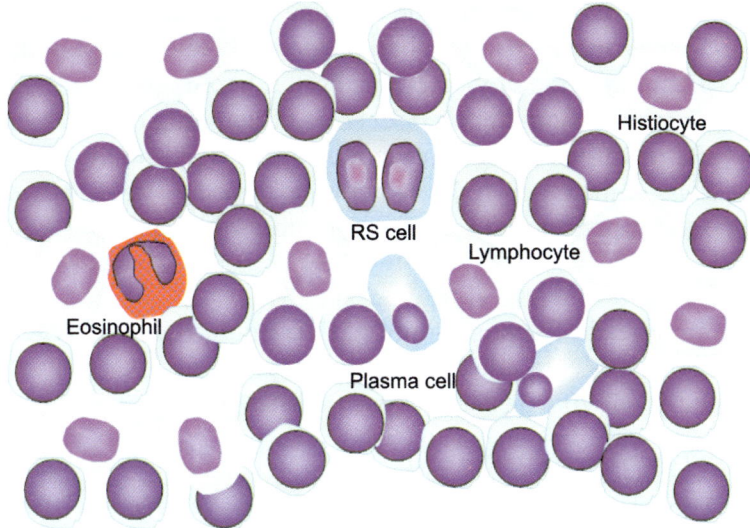

Fig. 18.2: Hodgkin's lymphoma

2. Mixed Cellularity

Frequent mononuclear and classical Reed-Sternberg cell are seen in the background of reactive cells composed of lymphocytes, macrophages and plasma cells (Fig. 18.2).

3. Lymphocytic Rich

Frequent mononuclear and classical Reed-Sternberg cell are seen in the background of lymphocyte rich reactive cells.

4. Lymphocytic Depleted

Reticular variant—Frequent L and H variant Reed-Sternberg cell are seen with paucity of background reactive cells.

Diffuse fibrosis variant—Classical Reed-Sternberg cell and variants are seen in the fibrillar background with few reactive cells.

Clinical Features

- Painless, nontender, discrete, rubbery lymph node enlargement
- Constitutional symptoms like fever, night sweats, and weight loss
- Cyclical pattern of fever (Pel-Ebstein fever) is rarely seen
- Cell mediated immunity is depressed

Staging of Hodgkin's Disease

Stage I	Single lymph node/region
Stage I E	Single extralymphatic region

Stage II	Two or more lymph node on same side of diaphragm
Stage II E	Two or more extralymphatic region on same side of diaphragm
Stage III	Lymphadenopathy on both sides of diaphragm
Stage III S	Lymphadenopathy on both sides of diaphragm with splenomegaly
Stage III E	Extralymphatic region on both sides of diaphragm
Stage IV	Disseminated or multiple nodal/extranodal sites involvement

Prefix 'A' is added for presence of systemic symptoms and 'B' for its absence.

Prognosis

Tumor stage is prognostically more important than morphological type.
- In Stage I and IIA 90% cure rate with treatment protocol
- In Stage III and IV 60–70% 5 years disease free survival

Non-Hodgkin's Lymphoma (NHL)

It is monoclonal neoplastic proliferation of lymphoid tissue which lack Reed-Sternberg cell. Most cases arise in lymph nodes but few may lake origin at extra nodal site, stomach being most common extranodal site. It is usually a disease of middle and elderly persons.

Etiopathogenesis

Various factors found to be associated with NHL are:

1. Infections

- Viral—EBV, HTLV type 1, HIV, Hepatitis C
- Bacterial—*Helicobacter pylori* in MALT lymphoma of stomach

2. Immunodeficiency Diseases

Ataxia telangiectasia AIDS, radiotherapy/chemotherapy induced immunosuppression.

3. Autoimmune Diseases

Sjögren's syndrome and rheumatoid arthritis.

4. Chemicals and Drugs

Phenytoin, pesticides and anticancer drugs.

5. Cytogenetic Abnormality

Over expression of BCL-2 protein.

Classification

Various classifications are:
- Rappaport

- Lukes-Collins
- Working formulation for clinical usage
- Revised European-American lymphoid malignancy (REAL)
- WHO classification

Before REAL/WHO classification other classifications were based on light microscopic picture and do not correlate well with prognosis of disease. Therefore now updated REAL/WHO classification is used. It is based on cell lineage and morphology of cells and correlates well with clinical course of the disease.

REAL/WHO Classification of Lymphoid Neoplasm

B Cell Neoplasm

A. Precursor B Cell Neoplasm

1. B cell acute Lymphoblastic leukaemia/lymphoma (B-ALL)

B. Mature B Cell Neoplasm

1. B cell chronic lymphocytic leukaemia/small lymphocytic lymphoma
2. B-Prolymphocytic leukaemia
3. Lymphoplasmacytic lymphoma
4. Splenic marginal zone lymphoma
5. Hairy cell lymphoma
6. Plasma cell myeloma/plasmacytoma
7. Extranodal marginal B cell lymphoma of MALT type
8. Mantle cell lymphoma
9. Follicular lymphoma
10. Nodal marginal zone B cell lymphoma
11. Diffuse large B cell lymphoma
12. Burkitt's lymphoma

T cell and NK Neoplasm

A. Precursor T Cell Neoplasm

T Lymphoblastic lymphoma/leukaemia

B. Mature (Peripheral) T-cell Neoplasm

1. T cell prolymphocytic leukaemia
2. T cell granular lymphocytic leukaemia
3. Aggressive NK cell leukaemia
4. Adult T cell lymphoma/leukaemia
5. Extranodal NK/T cell lymphoma, nasal type
6. Enteropathy type T cell lymphoma
7. Hepatosplenic gamma/delta T cell lymphoma

8. Subcutaneous panniculitis like T cell lymphoma
9. Mycosis fungoides/Sézari syndrome
10. Anaplastic large cell lymphoma, primary cutaneous type
11. Peripheral T cell lymphoma, unspecified
12. Angioimmunoblastic T cell lymphoma
13. Anaplastic large cell lymphoma, primary systemic type

Morphological Features

Gross Features

- Group of enlarged lymph nodes appear matted
- On cutting it shows fish flesh like appearance

Microscopic Features

B cell lymphoid neoplasm

1. B Cell Acute Lymphoblastic Leukaemia/Lymphoma (B-ALL)

- Nodal architecture is completely effaced
- Neoplastic tissue is composed of lymphoblasts
- Lymphoblasts show large nucleus, condensed chromatin
- Nuclear membrane is convoluted/ cleaved with inconspicuous nucleoli
- Lymphoblasts are TdT (Terminal deoxynucleotidyl transferase) and CD-19 positive

2. B Cell Chronic Lymphocytic Leukaemia/Small Lymphocytic Lymphoma

- Chronic lymphocytic leukaemia is present in peripheral blood
- Small lymphocytic lymphoma is a disease of lymph nodes
- Pancytopaenia is seen when bone marrow is involved
- Lymph node shows effacement of nodal architecture composed of sheets of mature cells (Fig. 18.3)

3. Follicular Lymphoma

Effacement of nodal architecture, composed of centrocytic cells in follicular pattern.

4. Mantle Cell Lymphoma

- Diffuse nodular pattern of effacement by mantle cell
- Mantle cells show irregular nucleus with inconspicuous nucleoli

5. Diffuse Large Cells Lymphoma

Complete effacement of nodal architecture composed of centroblasts and immunoblasts.

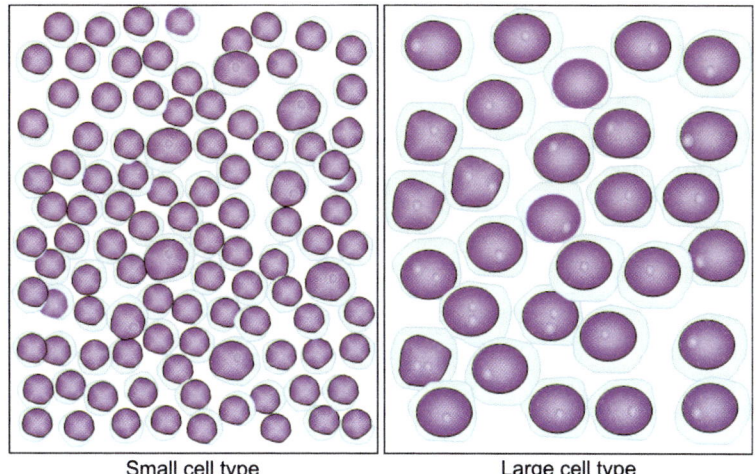

Small cell type   Large cell type

Fig. 18.3: Non-Hodgkin's lymphoma

6. Burkitt's Lymphoma

- Usually children are affected with extranodal site involvement like maxilla/ mandible in African type, abdominal viscera in American type
- High degree of mitoses creates characteristic starry sky appearance

7. MALT Lymphoma (Mucosa Associated Lymphoid Tissue)

- Arise in MALT like salivary gland, GIT, lungs, orbit, and breast
- It is seen in elderly persons

T cell Lymphoid Neoplasm

1. Precursor T cell Malignancy (T-ALL/Lymphoma)

- Similar to B cell ALL/lymphoma
- T Lymphoblasts are TdT positive CD-27 positive

2. Mycosis Fungoides/Sézary Syndrome

- Cutaneous T cell lymphoma characterized by infiltration of epidermis and dermis by neoplastic T cells (cells with cerebriform nucleus)
- Its Leukaemic phase is called Sézary syndrome resulting in appearance of neoplastic cells in blood

3. Adult T cell Lymphoma/Leukaemia

Lymph nodes, liver, spleen, skin, is infiltrated by mature lymphocytes. If cells appear in peripheral blood, it is called chronic lymphocytic leukaemia.

4. Peripheral T-cell Lymphoma

Usually young adults are affected. It consists of four types
• Angioimmunoblastic type
• Extranodal lymphoma of nasal type
• T cell lymphoma of enteropathic type
• T cell lymphoma of hepatosplenic type

Laboratory Diagnosis

1. Anaemia of normocytic, normochromic type
2. Bone marrow involvement causes pancytopaenia, leukoerythroblastic picture
3. NHL may be converted into leukaemic phase
4. Hypreuricemia, hypercalcaemia

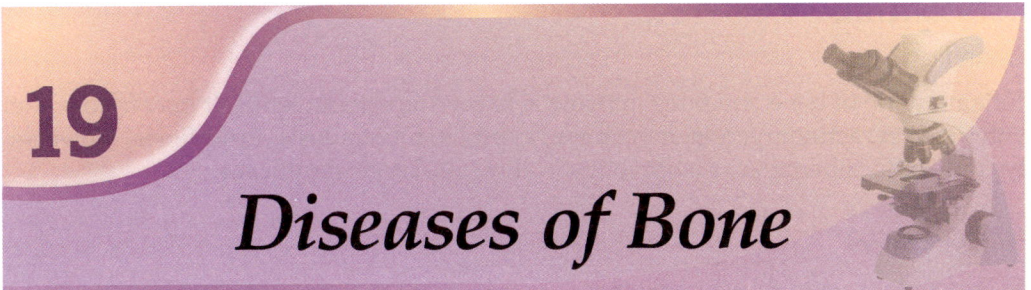

Diseases of Bone

DEFINITION

Skeletal system consists of bone and cartilage. Bones provide mechanical support and act as mineral reservoir of calcium. Role of cartilage is in the growth and repair of bone and smooth movement of joints.

Components of Bone

- **Outer cortical** or compact part provides structural rigidity to the body. It is composed of mineralized collagen traversed by concentric osteocytic lacunae surrounding blood vessels (haversian canal).
- **Inner trabecular** or cancellous bone traverses the marrow space. It maintains calcium homeostasis.

Histological Features

Bone

- **Osteoblasts** are new bone forming cells; its activity is reflected by alkaline phosphatase level in plasma.
- **Osteocytes** are osteoblasts which get incorporated in bone matrix.
  - In woven bone they are closely packed and numerous in number.
  - In lamellar bone osteocytes are fewer in number separated by collagen bundles.
- **Osteoclasts** are multinucleated cells responsible for resorption of bone. Its activity is reflected by acid phosphatase level in blood.
- **Bone matrix** is composed of mineralized collagen type I.

Cartilage

- Cartilage lacks blood vessels, lymphatics and nerves.
- **Matrix** is composed of collagen type II and proteoglycans with high water content. Fibro cartilage contain abundant collagen bundle while elastic cartilage contain abundant elastic fibers.
- **Chondrocytes** are derived from chondroblasts.

OSTEOMYELITIS

Definition

Inflammation of bone and bone marrow is known as osteomyelitis. It may follow after enteric fever, actinomycosis, mycetoma, syphilis, tuberculosis, brucellosis. However, bacterial and tubercular osteomyelitis is clinically more significant.

Classification

1. Pyogenic (bacterial) osteomyelitis
2. Tubercular osteomyelitis
3. Syphilitic osteomyelitis

Pyogenic Osteomyelitis

Bacterial infections to bone and marrow occurs due to

- Haematogenous spread through bacteraemia, septicemia, and pyaemia
- Direct extension from adjacent area like jaw and skull
- As complication of compound fracture, surgical procedures, debility and immuno-suppression

Etiology

- Most common organism (80–90%) is *Staphylococcus aureus*
- Less common are *Streptococci, E. coli, Pseudomonas,* and *Klebsiella*, Anaerobes

Location

Most frequent sites are areas of rapid growth where vascularity is high, like distal femur, proximal tibia, proximal humerus and distal radius.

Clinical Features

Pain and tenderness at local site, fever and malaise

Stages of Infections

a. Localization of bacteria is influenced by vascularity and velocity of circulation. Highly vascular areas with slow circulation are prone to get infected.
b. Induction of inflammation and edema, raising tissue pressure in bone.
c. Infection passes via Haversian system to periosteum leading to subperiosteal abscess (Brodie's abscess).
d. Lifting of periosteum impairs blood supply; hence bone is devitalized resulting in to sequestrum formation. Reactive bone deposited around living tissue is known as involucrum (Fig. 19.1).
e. Rupture of periosteum leads to development of discharging sinus.

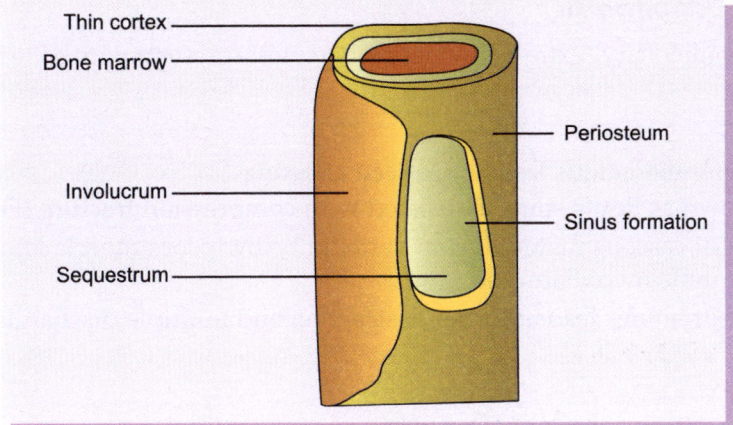

Fig. 19.1: Chronic osteomyelitis

Morphological Changes

Acute Osteomyelitis

• **Suppuration**—Collection of neutrophilic exudate and amorphous debris.

Chronic Osteomyelitis

• **Sequestrum** formation—Necrosed thin cortical bone, due to ischaemic necrosis.
• **Neo osteogenesis**—New bone formation beneath the periosteum and around necrosed bone known as **Involucrum.**

Osteomyelitis of Garre

Long-standing neo-osteogenesis leads to sclerotic pattern of osteomyelitis called chronic non suppurative osteosclerotic or **osteomyelitis of Garre**.

Brodie's Abscess

Occasionally acute osteomyelitis may be walled off by fibrous tissue and granulation tissue known as **Brodie's abscess.**

Laboratory Investigations

• Complete blood cell count shows neutrophilic leukocytosis.
• X-ray shows bone destruction.

Complications

1. Septicemia which may lead to endocarditis
2. Acute bacterial arthritis
3. Pathological fracture
4. Squamous cell carcinoma in long-standing cases

Tubercular Osteomyelitis

About 1–3% pulmonary/extra pulmonary tuberculosis presents with bone involvement.

Location

Tubercular granulomatous lesions are seen affecting
- Spine, known as Pott's spine associated with compression fracture (Fig. 19.2)
- Collection of caseous material from vertebra below psoas muscle known as psoas abscess or lumbar cold abscess
- Bones of extremities leads to bone destruction and multiple discharging sinus

Mode of Spread

- Haematogenous
- Direct invasion
- Lymphatics

Clinical Features

Pain, fever, weight loss

Morphological Features

- Tubercular lesions consist of central caseative necrosis with chronic granulomatous foci destroying the bone forming multiple discharging sinuses through muscle and skin.

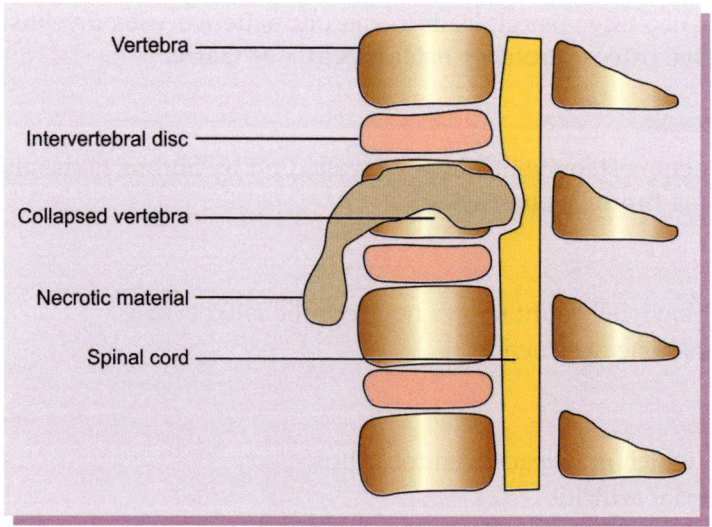

Fig. 19.2: Pott's spine

- Involvement of vertebrae leads to compression fracture and destruction of intervertebral disc. Extension of caseous material and pus from lumbar vertebrae to the sheath of psoas muscle produce psoas abscess.

Complications

1. Psoas abscess
2. Fracture
3. Neurological manifestations
4. Tubercular arthritis
5. Sinus formation
6. Ankylosis

FRACTURE HEALING (Fig. 19.3)

Fracture healing depends on
- Type of fracture, traumatic/pathological
- Complete/incomplete
- Simple/comminuted/compound

1. Primary Union

When broken ends are approximated and aligned properly, fracture heals by medullary callous formation without periosteal callous formation.

2. Secondary Union

When there is gap between broken ends, fracture heals by secondary union. Secondary union involves following steps.

A. Procallous Formation

- Haematoma forms loose meshwork of granulation tissue
- Macrophages clear local inflammatory exudate, debris and necrosed bone
- Soft tissue callous is formed by ingrowths of granulation tissue
- Inner layer of periosteum lay down the osteoid matrix/chondroid matrix
- Osteoid/chondroid matrix undergo calcification forming woven bone callous

B. Osseous Callous Formation

- Woven bone is cleared by osteoclasts
- Osteoblasts and new blood vessel invade procallous
- Osteoid tissue is laid down by osteoblast which is calcified
- Calcified lamellar bone is formed in the scaffolding of procallous

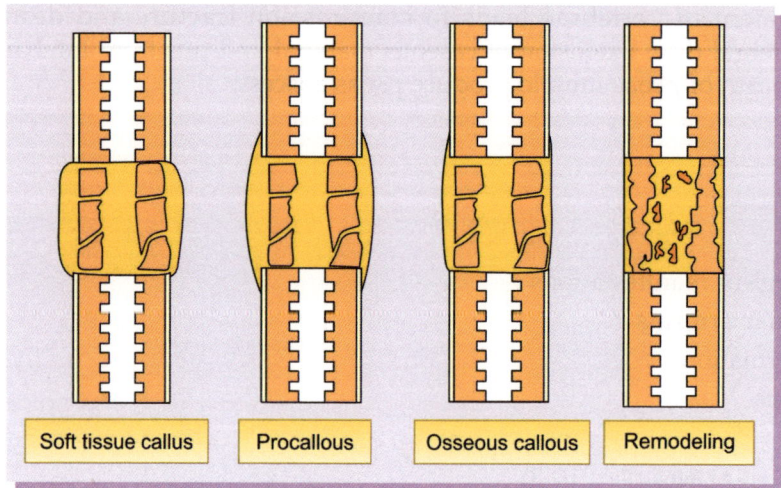

| Soft tissue callus | Procallous | Osseous callous | Remodeling |

Fig. 19.3: Fracture healing

C. Remodeling

- Shape of newly formed bone is modified by osteoblastic and osteoclastic activity
- External callous is cleared away and compact bone is formed in intermediate callous
- Bone marrow develops in internal callous

Complications

Fibrous Union

If immobilization is not done properly, bone get united by fibrous tissue forming false joint at fractured site (pseudoarthrosis)

Nonunion

If soft tissue is interposed between fractured ends, non union results.

Delayed Union

Factors causing delayed healing are infections, poor nutrition, movement, old age, etc.

DISORDERS OF BONE GROWTH AND DEVELOPMENT

1. *Local disorders:* It includes one bone or group of bone presenting as absence, diminished, fused with other bone or extra bones. For example, syndactyly (two digits fused together) supernumerary (extra rib)
2. *Systemic disorders:* Disorders which involves bone growth and development

Achondroplasia (Dwarfism)

It is autosomal dominant disorder.

Defect

It involves selective interference with normal endochondral ossification at cartilaginous growth plate of long bones.

Effects

- Long bones become short
- Skull grows normally

Osteogenesis Imperfecta

It is autosomal dominant or recessive disorder.

Defect

Disorder of Type I collagen synthesis

Effects

- Thin and non existent cortex results in fragile bones which are liable to get fractured easily. It may become evident at birth (osteogenesis imperfecta congenita) or may become evident during adolescence (osteogenesis imperfecta tarda)
- Extra skeletal manifestations are blue transparent sclera, hearing loss due to bone abnormality of inner and middle ear, imperfect teeth

Osteopetrosis

It is autosomal dominant or recessive disorder.

Defect

Failure of normal osteoclastic function

Effects

- Increased skeletal mass but susceptible to get fractured
- Obliteration of marrow manifests as anaemia, neutropenia, thrombocytopaenia, hepatosplenomegaly, due to extramedullary erythropoiesis
- Obliteration of neural canal leads to hydrocephalous, neurological manifestations, deafness and blindness

METABOLIC AND ENDOCRINE BONE DISORDERS

1. Osteoporosis
2. Osteomalacia and rickets

3. Scurvy
4. Osteitis fibrosa cystica and osteoporosis due to hyperthyroidism
5. Cretinism due to hypothyroidism
6. Gigantism, acromegaly and dwarfism due to pituitary dysfunction
7. Renal dystrophy due to chronic renal failure

Osteoporosis

There is quantitative reduction in bone tissue mass resulting in fragile bones.

A. *Primary Osteoporosis*

- Idiopathic type is seen in young persons
- Involutional type is seen in postmenopausal women and elderly persons
- Exact cause is not known but possibly due to increased osteoclastic activity and decreased osteoblastic activity.

Risk factors for primary osteoporosis are
- White and female are at more risk than black and male
- Reduced physical activity
- Deficiency of estrogen in female and deficiency of androgens in male
- Hyperparathyroidism
- Deficiency of calcitonin and estrogen
- Deficiency of vitamin D

B. *Secondary Osteoporosis*

It is secondary to some other causes like
- Immobilization
- Chronic anaemia
- Hepatic disease
- Starvation
- Drugs

Morphological Features

- Thinning of cortex and enlargement of medullary cavity
- In active osteoporosis turn over is increased, i.e. osteoclasts are numerous as well as osteoblast are also increased in number. Width of osteoid seam is normal.
- In inactive osteoporosis, turnover is reduced, i.e. decreased osteoclasts with normal or decreased osteoblasts. Width of osteoid seam is normal or reduced.

Clinical Features

- Common in elderly persons, more common in postmenopausal women

- Fragile bones are associated with increased risk of fracture, pain and deformity
- Patient may be asymptomatic or complains of backache

Laboratory Tests

- Radiological evidences are apparent when more than 30% reduction of bone mass occurred
- Serum calcium, phosphorus and alkaline phosphatase are normal

Osteitis Fibrosa Cystica (Brown tumor)

Primary or secondary hyperparathyroidism results in increased osteolytic activity which cause increased bone resorption. Severe and prolonged hyperparathyroidism leads to osteitis fibrosa cystica.

Clinical Features

- Increased susceptibility of fracture
- Skeletal deformity
- Joint pain and dysfunction of bone

Biochemical Alterations

- Parathyroid hormone level is increased
- Serum calcium is high
- Serum phosphorus is low
- Urinary excretion of calcium is increased

Morphological Features

Severity of lesion in long bone may vary from generalized rarefaction to cyst formation with destruction of bone.

Gross Features

- Focal area of cortical bone is eroded
- Loss of lamina dura occurs at the root of teeth

Microscopic Features

- **Rarefaction**—Earliest changes are increased bone resorption and demineralization at periosteal and endosteal surface of cortex.
- **Osteitis fibrosa**—Bone and bone marrow is replaced by fibrous tissue. Large numbers of osteoclasts are seen in trabecular and cortical bone.
- **Cystica**—Micro fractures and micro haemorrhage are seen in marrow leading to formation of cyst.
- **Brown tumor**—Haemosiderin laden macrophages are seen in haemorrhagic area producing brown color mass.

Paget's Disease (Osteitis deformans)

First time described by Sir James Paget in 1877. It is osteolytic and osteosclerotic disease of bone affecting predominantly male of more than 50 years age.

Types

- Involving one bone (monostotic)
- Involving many bones (polystotic)

Etiology

- Unknown
- Evidences suggest possibility of paramyxoma viral infection or genetic autosomal dominant disorder

Clinical Features

- Monostotic are asymptomatic
- Polystotic may present with pain, fracture, deformity and occasionally sarcoma

Morphological Features

- Order of bone involvement in monostotic form is **tibia**, pelvis, femur, skull and vertebrae
- Order of bone involvement in polystotic form is **vertebrae**, pelvis, femur, skull and tibia

Stages of Paget's Disease

  I. **Osteolytic stage**—Large number of osteoclasts cause bone resorption
 II. **Mixed stage**—Mosaic pattern of osteoblastic and osteoclastic activity is seen
III. **Quiescent stage**—After long duration compact and sclerotic bone is formed, but it is poorly mineralized and soft. Radiologically cotton wool appearance is seen

TUMOR LIKE LESIONS OF BONE

These are non neoplastic conditions resembling neoplasm.

Fibrous Dysplasia

It is developmental defect of bone characterized by localized area of replacement of bone by fibrous tissue, composed of trabeculae of woven bone in whorled fibrous tissue. Radiologically well demarcated ground glass appearance is seen.

Types

1. Monostotic
   - It is most common type of fibrous dysplasia. Lesions affect solitary bone

- Commonly patients of 20–30 years age group are affected
- Order of bones involved is ribs, craniofacial, femur, tibia and humerus
- Usually remain asymptomatic, infrequently produce tumor-like mass

2. Polystotic
   - Several bones are affected at a time
   - Usually seen in less than 20 years age group
   - Order of bones involved is craniofacial, ribs, vertebrae, and long bones

3. Albright's syndrome
   - Polystotic fibrous dysplasia is associated with endocrine dysfunction
   - Endocrine dysfunctions present as skin pigmentation, sexual precocity and others symptoms
   - Commonly females are affected
   - Accounts for less than 5% cases of fibrous dysplasia

Gross Features

- Sharply demarcated localized mass with thin overlying cortex
- Cancellous bone is replaced by soft rubbery tissue with areas of haemorrhage and cyst formation

Microscopic Features

Benign fibroblastic tissue in whorled pattern with irregular curved trabeculae of woven bone and numerous osteoclasts

Fibrous Cortical Defect

- Metaphyseal cortex of long bone of children are involved
- Most commonly tibia and femur
- Generally solitary, sometimes multiple and bilaterally symmetrical lesion

Clinical Features

Patient is usually asymptomatic. X-ray shows eccentric lesion in metaphysis

Pathogenesis

Possibly as the result of some developmental defect in epiphyseal plate or possibly a tumor of histiocytic origin

Gross Features

Small brown granular mass less than 4 cm.

Microscopic Features

Fibrous tissue in storiform pattern with osteoclasts and focal areas of haemosiderin laden macrophages and foam cells

CYSTIC LESIONS OF BONE

Simple Solitary Bone Cyst

It is seen in children and adolescents, usually in metaphysis of upper end of humerus or femur

Gross Features

Cyst filled with clear fluid, thinning the cortex

Microscopic Features

Cyst wall is composed of fibro collagenous tissue with scattered osteoclasts and neoosteogenesis. Fracture may alter the appearance with secondary haemorrhage and haemosiderin laden macrophages.

Aneurysmal Bone Cyst

It is an expending osteolytic lesion filled with blood in metaphysis of long bone. Commonly seen in less than 30 years of age.

Gross Features

Large haemorrhagic mass covered by thin reactive bone

Microscopic Features

Cyst wall is composed of osteoid tissue with osteoclasts and endothelial lining

Ganglion Cyst

Usually seen in middle are group, commonly in lower end of humerus or lower end of tibia.

Gross Features

Multiloculated cyst filled with mucous. X-ray shows well-defined osteolytic area

Microscopic Features

Cyst wall is not lined by synovial tissue, but dense edematous connective tissue.

BONE TUMORS

Primary tumors involving bones are:

Histological type	Benign	Malignant
Haematopoietic (40%)	-	Myeloma
		Malignant lymphoma
Chondrogenic (22%)	Enchondroma	Chondrosarcoma
	Osteochondroma	Dedifferentiated chondrosarcoma
	Chondromyxoid fibroma	Mesenchymal chondrosarcoma
Osteogenic (20%)	Osteoma	Osteosarcoma
	Osteoid osteoma	
	Osteoblastoma	
Unknown origin (10%)	Giant cell tumor	Ewing's sarcoma
		Malignant giant cell tumor
		Adamantinoma
Histiocytic origin	Fibrous histiocytoma	Malignant fibrous histiocytoma
Fibrogenic	Metaphyseal fibrous defect	Desmoplastic fibroma
		Fibrosarcoma
Notocordal	-	Chordoma
Vascular	Haemangioma	Haemangioendothelioma
		Haemangiopericytoma
Lipogenic	Lipoma	Liposarcoma

BONE FORMING TUMORS (OSTEOBLASTIC TUMORS)

Osteoblastic tumors are characterized by synthesis of osteoid/bone tissue by the tumor cells. There is no evidence of endochondral or reactive bone formation.

1. Osteoma

Bones Involved

Flat bones of skull and face, paranasal sinuses. Following trauma, subperiosteal haematoma or focal inflammation.

Clinical Features

- Commonly seen in middle age group
- Solitary and slow growing
- Present as deformity, obstruct sinus cavity, impinges on brain or eye

Gross Features

Sessile round or oval mass, projecting from surface

Microscopic Features

Tumor is composed of well-differentiated mature lamellar bone.

2. Osteoid Osteoma

Bones Involved

Long bones (femur, tibia), intracortical, occasionally intramedullary

Clinical Features

- Commonly seen in the 10–30 age group
- Present as intense local pain responding to aspirin, swelling and tenderness
- X-ray shows nidus <1.5 cm. Surrounded by sclerotic bone

Gross Features

Well-defined rounded to oval mass of <2 cm in size

Microscopic Features

Trabeculae of osteoid tissue rimmed by osteoblasts, separated by vascularised stroma, enveloped by sclerotic bone.

3. Osteoblastoma

Bones Involved

Vertebrae, metaphysis of tibia, femur, humerus, pelvis. May be intracortical or intramedullary.

Clinical Features

- Commonly seen in the 10–30 age group
- Present as dull aching pain not responding to aspirin

Gross Features

Larger than 2 cm rounded, oval mass

Microscopic Features

- Calcified osteoid tissue growing within highly vascularised connective tissue
- Sclerosis is minimal

4. Osteosarcoma

Osteosarcoma is malignant mesenchymal tumor producing osteoid tissue, is most common malignant tumor after myeloma and lymphoma.

Bones Involved

Metaphysis of long bones, order of frequency is lower end of femur, upper end of tibia, upper end of humerus. Usually intramedullary in origin (Fig. 19.4).

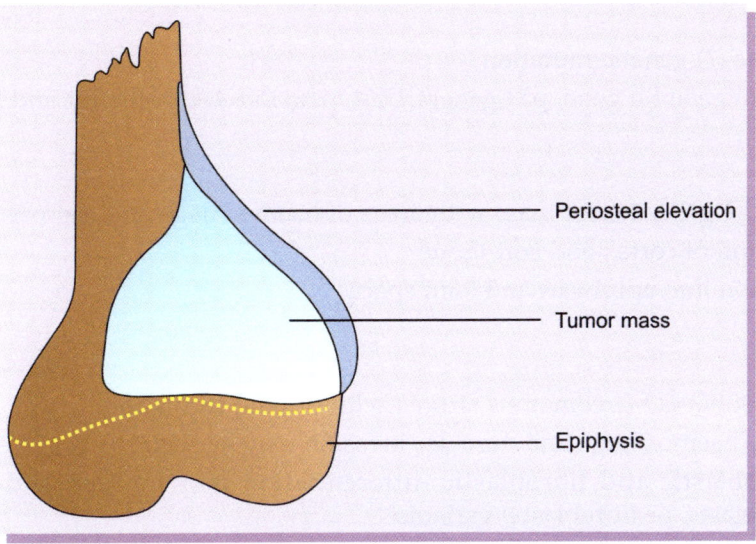

Periosteal elevation

Tumor mass

Epiphysis

Fig. 19.4: Osteosarcoma

Clinical Features

- Progressive painful enlargement of bone
- Pathological fracture
- X-ray shows large destructive mixed density mass with irregular infiltrative radiating margins (Sun burst appearance)
- Tumor breaks through the cortex inducing periosteal bone formation which lifts the periosteum. Triangular shadow between cortex and raised periosteum is called Codman's triangle.

Classification

1. Primary osteosarcoma—arise *de novo*
2. Secondary osteosarcoma—arise secondary to pre-existing disease like
   - Paget's disease
   - Fibrous dysplasia
   - Osteochondroma
   - Enchondroma
   - Bone infarct
   - Chronic osteomyelitis
   - Radiation exposure
   - Chemotherapy

Pathogenesis

- Idiopathic (?) genetic mutation
- Abnormal gene Rb gene, p53 gene, CDK4, p16, INK4A, cyclin D1 and MDM2

Gross Features

- Gray white gritty tumor mass with areas of haemorrhage and necrosis
- Destruction of cortex and soft tissue
- Penetration into epiphysis and joint space

Microscopic Features

- Undifferentiated/sarcomatous stroma with osteoid formation
- Necrosis, haemorrhage and vascular invasion may be seen
- Chondroblastic and fibroblastic differentiation may be seen and labeled as chondroblastic or fibroblastic variants

Topographical Variants

1. Juxtacortical (parosteal)
   - Seen in old age, located on posterior aspect of femur
   - Low-grade tumor encircling the bone with good prognosis
2. Periosteal osteosarcoma
   - Growth is seen over the surface of cortex, predominantly chondroblastic
   - High-grade tumor with poor prognosis
3. Osteosarcoma of jaw
   - Seen in older age at mandible and maxilla
   - Chondroblastic with good prognosis

Metastasis

Osteosarcoma metastasize to lungs, other bones, pleura, heart

Diagnosis

- Fine needle aspiration cytology (FNAC)
- Biopsy for histopathological examination

CARTILAGE FORMING TUMORS (CHONDROBLASTIC TUMORS)

Cartilaginous tumors are characterized by hyaline or myxoid cartilage formation

1. Osteochondroma (Exostosis)

It may be multiple hereditary or sporadic solitary

Bones Involved

Metaphysis of lower end of femur, upper tibia, upper humerus

Clinical Features

- Commonly seen in adolescent and young adults
- Asymptomatic or present as pain with deformity
- X-ray shows metaphyseal lesion growing in direction opposite to adjacent joint

Gross Features

Sessile or pedunculated shape with narrow base in continuity with cortex covered by cartilaginous cap (Fig. 19.5)

Microscopic Features

Inner lamellar bone and bone marrow covered by hyaline cartilage

2. Chondroma

Bones Involved

Commonly short bones of hand and foot are involved

Topographical Types

- Intramedullary (enchondroma)
- Subperiosteal

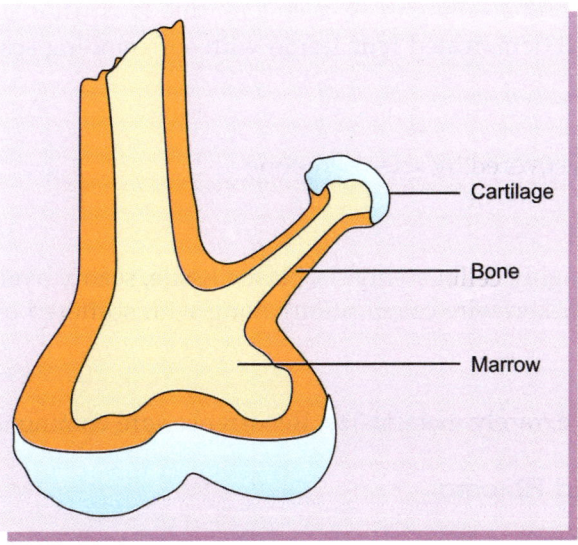

Fig. 19.5: Exostosis (osteochondroma)

Types Based on Numbers

- Solitary chondroma
- Multiple chondroma, i.e. enchondromatosis, nonhereditary (Ollier's disease)
- Multiple chondromas with soft tissue haemangioma, hereditary (Maffucci's syndrome)

Clinical Features

- Common between 20 and 50 years of age
- Mostly asymptomatic occasionally painful and with pathological fracture

Gross Features

Bluish gray transparent, lobulated mass, usually smaller than 3 cm

Microscopic Features

It is composed of mature hyaline cartilage separated by vascularised fibrous tissue

3. Chondroblastoma

Bones Involved

It involves epiphysis of lower end of femur, upper end of tibia, upper end of humerus

Clinical Features

- Usually males less than 20 years are affected
- Present with painful swelling or swollen joint due to effusion in adjoining joint
- X-ray shows well demarcated lytic lesion with surrounding sclerosis

Gross Features

Well-defined mass covered by sclerosed bone

Microscopic Features

It is composed of highly cellular chondroblastic tissue, scanty hyaline matrix and foci of calcification (Chicken wire calcification) along with scattered osteoclasts.

Prognosis

It is locally invasive, rarely metastasize. Recurrences are common.

4. Chondromyxoid Fibroma

Bones Involved

Metaphysis of upper end of tibia, lower end of femur

Clinical Features
- Young adults are affected
- Present with localized dull aching pain
- X-ray shows large sharply outlined area surrounded by sclerosed bone

Gross Features
Solid glistening lobulated soft to firm mass of 3–8 cm in size

Microscopic Features
It is composed of less cellular myxoid tissue separated by fibrous tissue and nodules of poorly formed hyaline cartilage. Small foci of calcification and osteoclasts may be seen.

5. Chondrosarcoma
It is malignant neoplasm of chondrocytes.

Bones Involved
Arise from medullary cavity of long bones, pelvis, costochondral junction of ribs and shoulder.

Clinical Features
- Commonly seen in the 30–60 age group
- Slowly growing mass, presents with pain
- X-ray shows expansile osteolytic growth with foci of calcification

Morphological Classification
1. Chondrosarcoma (hyaline/myxoid)
2. Clear cell chondrosarcoma
3. Dedifferentiated chondrosarcoma
4. Mesenchymal chondrosarcoma

Topographic Classification
- Intramedullary
  - Central skeleton—pelvis, ribs, shoulder
  - Peripheral skeleton—long bones
- Juxtacortical

Gross Features
- Large bulky translucent lobulated firm mass with foci of calcification
- On cutting gray white gelatinous appearance

Microscopic Features

Lobules of malignant chondrocytes (plump hyperchromatic multilobated two or more nuclei with two or more cells in one lacunae) with abundant mitoses are seen along with necrosis and foci of calcification.

GIANT CELL TUMOR (OSTEOCLASTOMA)

Bones Involved

Epiphysis of long bones, lower end of femur, upper end of tibia, lower end of radius, upper end of fibula.

Clinical Features

- Common age group is 20–40, predominantly male
- Present with pain, swelling, pathological fracture
- X-ray shows osteolytic lesion without peripheral sclerosis, destroying cortex with soap bubble appearance

Gross Features

Well circumscribed solid dark brown mass. On cutting haemorrhage and necrosis is seen.

Microscopic Features

It is composed of stromal cells and multinucleated giant cells along with haemorrhage and necrosis. Focal areas of osteoid tissue may be seen. Stromal cells are neoplastic element and correlate well with clinical outcome of tumor.

EWING'S SARCOMA

It is highly malignant small cell tumor.

Bones Involved

It arise from medullary cavity of diaphysis and metaphysis of long bones (femur, tibia, humerus, fibula) and flat bones (pelvis and scapula)

Clinical Features

- Children and young adults of 5–20 age group are affected
- Present with pain, tenderness, swelling, with fever
- X-ray shows reactive periosteal bone formation around osteolytic lesion (onion skin appearance)

Classification

1. Classical (skeletal) Ewing's sarcoma

2. Soft tissue sarcoma
3. Primitive neuroectodermal tumor (PNET)
   Chromosomal abnormality is reciprocal translocation t (11; 22) (q24; q12)

Morphological Features

It arise from (?) endothelial/pericyte/bone marrow/mesenchymal tissue.

Gross Features

Gray white lobular soft friable mass

Microscopic Features

Small rounded monotonous cells with uniform nuclei are seen in nests and lobules separated by fibrovascular septa. Tumor cells form pseudo rosettes around blood vessels with necrosis away from blood vessels.

Prognosis

- Early metastasis to lung, liver bones and brain is seen
- With combined chemotherapy and radiotherapy outcome is good

CHORDOMA

It is a slow growing malignant tumor from remnants of notochord (primitive axial skeleton) normally present in nucleus pulposus of vertebral body.

Bones Involved

Axial skeleton (sacral and sphenooccipital)

Clinical Features

- Commonly seen > 40 years of age
- Present with symptoms of cord compression

Gross Features

Soft lobulated translucent gelatinous mass with haemorrhage

Microscopic Features

Nests of vacuolated physaliphorus cells are seen in mucoid background material.

METASTATIC BONE TUMORS

Characteristic Features

- These are more frequent than primary bone tumors

- Most of them come through haematogenous spread
- Foci of metastasis may be single or multiple
- X-ray shows osteolytic lesions

Primary Tumor

Carcinoma metastasis is more common than sarcoma, to the bone, e.g.

Carcinoma From

- Breast, prostate, testis
- Lung, kidney, stomach
- Thyroid, cervix, uterus, urinary bladder
- Melanoma, neuroblastoma, etc.

Sarcoma From

Alveolar and embryonal rhabdomyosarcoma

20

Diseases of Oral Cavity

Developmental Anomalies

1. **Facial cleft**—Upper cleft lip and cleft palate occurs because of failure of fusion of facial processes.
2. **Fordyce's granules**—Under developed sebaceous glands appear as yellow spots on lip and buccal mucosa.
3. **Leukoedema**—Asymptomatic gray white patches appear on buccal mucosa due to intracellular edema.
4. **Developmental defect of tongue**—Microglossia, macroglossia, fissured tongue, bifid tongue, tongue tie, hairy tongue.

Mucocutaneous Lesions

A. Lichen Planus

- Oral lichen planus is a chronic condition, characterized by interlacing network of white areas inside oral cavity.
- Histological characteristic features are marked hyperkeratosis, focal hypergranulosis; saw toothed rete ridges and basal layer dyskeratosis.
- In dermis band like mononuclear infiltrate are seen.

B. Vesicular Lesions

Vesicles or bullous lesions seen over the oral mucosa are:

Pemphigus Vulgaris

Vesicular eruption filled with serum and acantholytic cells, occurs due suprabasal cleavage of epidermis.

Pemphigoid

Vesicle is formation occur due to subepidermal cleavage and no acantholytic cells are seen.

Erythema Multiforme

Vesicle is formed by subcorneal cleavage and filled with neutrophilic exudate.

Stevens-Johnson Syndrome

Severe and fatal form of erythema multiforme developed following ingestion of sulfa drugs.

Epidermolysis Bullosa

It is a hereditary condition with subepidermal bullae over skin and mucosa.

Inflammatory Diseases

1. Stomatitis

Inflammation of mucous membrane of mouth is called stomatitis. Various causes are:

a. Aphthous Ulcer

It is the commonest oral ulcerative lesion of unknown cause. It is often precipitated by emotional factors, stress, allergy, hormonal imbalance and nutritional deficiencies, gastrointestinal disturbances and trauma.

b. Herpetic Stomatitis

An acute illness seen in infants and young children is a manifestation of herpes simplex virus. Lesions are in the form of vesicles around lip.

c. Necrotizing Stomatitis

Commonly it is seen in poorly nourished children, immunodeficiency states and stressful conditions. The lesions show severe inflammatory necrosis of marginal gingiva extending to oral mucosa and cheek.

d. Mycotic

It is commonly due to actinomycosis and candidiasis; appear as opportunistic infection in immunocompromised patients.

2. Glossitis

Acute glossitis is seen in measles and scarlet fever. Chronic glossitis is seen in pellagra and other deficiency states of vitamin B. Chronic atrophic glossitis is seen in iron deficiency, pernicious anaemia characterized by smooth raw tongue with atrophied papillae.

3. Syphilitic Lesions

Extragenital primary lesion is seen on lips. Secondary lesions show maculopapular eruption in oral cavity. In tertiary syphilis gumma or diffuse fibrosis is seen in palate and tongue. Oral lesion of congenital syphilis is fissure at the angle of mouth and peg-shaped notched Hutchinson's incisors.

4. HIV Infection

Oral manifestations are opportunistic infections, malignancy, hairy leukoplakia and recurrent aphthous ulcers in mouth.

Tumor Like Lesions

1. Fibrous Growth

Fibrous growths in oral cavity are very common due to inflammation and chronic irritation. For example
- **Fibroepithelial polyp** is a fibrous growth covered by squamous epithelium, occurs due to chronic irritation/trauma.
- **Fibrous epulis** occurring over gingiva following trauma.
- **Denture hyperplasia** due to ill-fitting of denture.
- **Submucous fibrosis** is seen in person chewing tobacco, catechu and betel nut.

2. Pyogenic Granuloma

It is elevated bright red swelling on the lips, tongue, buccal mucosa, and gingiva. It is composed of fibrovascular proliferative tissue with inflammatory exudate.

3. Mucocele

It is a mucous filled cystic lesion occurring due to rupture of mucous glands. It elicits inflammation in the surrounding tissue. True epithelium is not evident.

4. Ranula

Ranula is large mucocele located on the floor of mouth, lined by true epithelium.

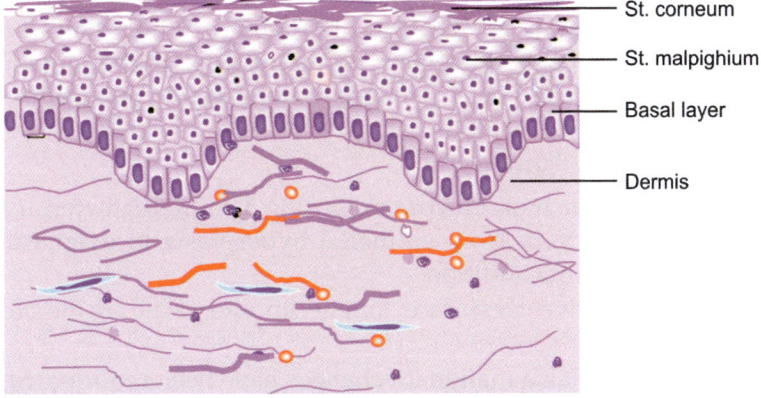

Fig. 20.1: Normal skin layer

5. *Dermoid Cyst*

It is tumor like cystic mass composed of stratified squamous epithelium enclosing keratinous debris. The cyst wall contain sebaceous and sweat glands and hair follicles.

Benign Tumors

A. *Squamous Papilloma*

It is characterized by finger like papillary projections over the surface. Microscopically papillae are composed of fibrovascular core covered by squamous epithelium.

B. *Haemangioma*

Haemangioma can occur any where in the mouth. Commonest form is capillary type, although cavernous and mixed type may also be seen. Lobules of proliferating capillaries are seen in capillary type lesion.

C. *Lymphangioma*

Most commonly seen on the tongue producing macroglossia, may also be seen on lips and cheek. Cystic hygroma is a peculiar form of lymphangioma occurring on lateral side of neck.

D. *Fibroma*

True fibroma is uncommon benign tumor in oral cavity. Most fibrous lesions found are fibrous growths.

E. *Fibromatosis Gingivae*

It is a fibrous overgrowth of unknown etiology occurring over gingiva.

F. *Tumors of Minor Salivary Gland (see in salivary gland)*

G. *Other Benign Tumors*

Granular cell myoblastoma is an unusual oral benign tumor seen in the tongue. Neurilemoma, neurofibroma, lipoma, giant cell granuloma, rhabdomyoma, osteoma, chondroma, plasmacytoma and naevi are rare tumors seen in oral cavity.

Premalignant Lesion (Leukoplakia)

- It is defined as white patch on mucosa exceeding 5 cm in diameter. It is epithelial thickening which may vary from epithelial hyperplasia to dysplasia, therefore classified as premalignant condition.
- Cheek, angle of mouth, alveolar surface, tongue, lip, and palate are the site commonly involved.
- In 4–6% cases of leukoplakia malignant changes have been reported. Speckled and nodular form is more liable to be converted into malignancy.

- Etiological factors responsible for the pathogenesis are heavy smoking, chronic irritation, and alcohol, hot and spicy food.

Gross Features

White patch with slightly elevated smooth or wrinkled surface over mucosa.

Microscopic Features

I. Hyperkeratotic Type

Epithelium show regular hyperplasia with hyperkeratosis (Fig. 20.2).

II. Dysplastic Type

- Epithelium shows irregular hyperplasia with loss of polarity and individual cell keratinization.
- Subepithelium shows mononuclear infiltrate composed of lymphocytes macrophages and plasma cells.
- Extent and degree of epithelial changes indicate severity of disease.
- Mild dysplasia reverts back to normal, while severe dysplasia may progress to malignancy.
- When dysplasia involves whole thickness of epidermis the condition is known as **carcinoma in situ** and my progress to invasive squamous cell carcinoma (Fig. 20.3).

Malignant Tumors

1. Squamous Cell Carcinoma

- It is most common malignant neoplasm of oral cavity. In India it is one of the common types of malignancy, because of tobacco and betel nut chewing habits.

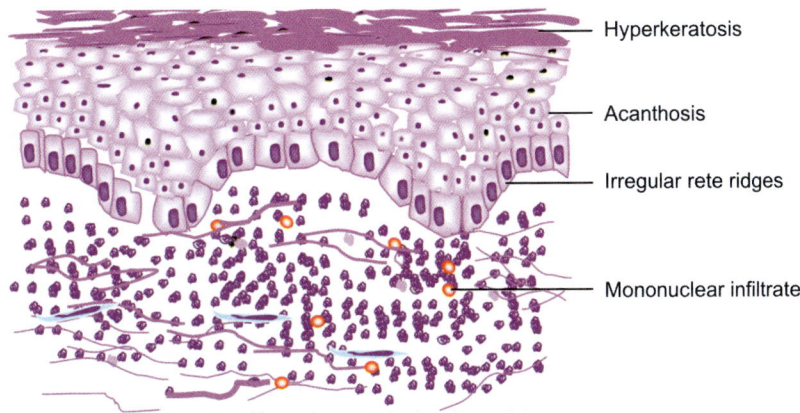

Fig. 20.2: Hyperkeratotic leukoplakia

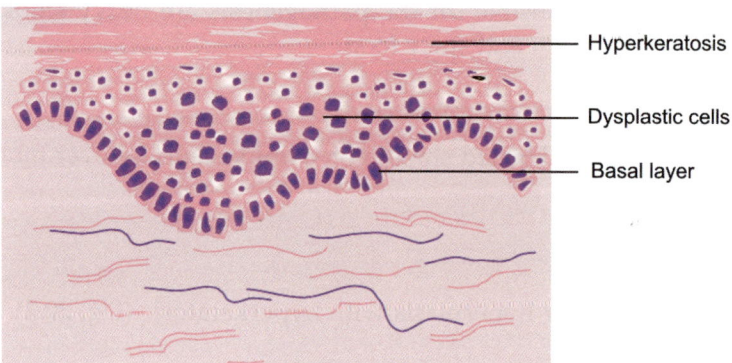

Fig. 20.3: Dysplasia

- Sites commonly involved are lips, tongue, buccal mucosa, alveolar-lingual sulcus, palate, floor of mouth
- Etiological factors are tobacco, alcohol, chronic irritation by ill-fitted dentures, chilies, poor oral hygiene, and HPV infection and radiation exposure.

Gross Features

Lesion may be ulcerative (most frequent), verrucous (wart like), nodular or hard scirrhous type.

Microscopic Features

Nests and masses of well differentiated to poorly differentiated malignant squamous epithelial cells are seen.

2. Other Malignant Tumors

Melanoma, lymphoma, malignant tumors of minor salivary glands and various sarcomas are quite uncommon tumors.

TEETH AND PERIODONTAL DISEASES

Dental Caries

It is characterized by destruction of calcified tissue of teeth.

Etiopathogenesis

Refined carbohydrate when react with saliva and acidogenic bacteria of mouth (streptococci) it produces organic acid which decalcify enamel and dentine. Enamel is composed of inorganic material which disintegrates easily. Dentine contain organic material also which is lysed by proteolytic enzymes produced by bacteria.

Morphological Features

- Caries occurs mainly at occlusal pits and fissures of molar and premolar teeth
- Earliest changes are chalky white spot on enamel which subsequently become yellow or brown and break down to form carious cavity, eventually cavity become larger. Once lesion reaches to dentine, it also begins to disintegrate.

Microscopic Features

Inflammation and necrosis of pulp is seen along with secondary dentine formation.

Complication of Dental Caries

- Acute and chronic pulpitis
- Apical granuloma, spread of infection around root of tooth may lead to granuloma formation
- Apical abscess, pus formation may occur in granuloma, which may further propagate to bone and results in cerebral abscess, meningitis, or cavernous sinus thrombosis

Periodontal Diseases

Chronic inflammation and degeneration of supporting tissue of teeth results in loss of tooth.

Etiology

- Leukaemia and scurvy are associated gingival swelling
- Pregnancy, puberty, drugs (Dilantin) are associated with gingivitis
- Chronic marginal gingivitis occur secondary to bacterial plaque, impacted food, diabetes, tooth decay, ill-fitting dentures

Microscopic Features

Heavy chronic inflammatory infiltrate, destruction of collagen and epithelial hyperplasia are seen.

EPITHELIAL CYSTS OF JAW

A. Inflammatory Cysts (Radicular cyst/Apical/Periodontal/Dental cyst)

Etiopathogenesis

It develops as a consequence of inflammation following destruction of dental pulp. Pulpitis and apical granuloma develops. The epithelial cells of Mallasez present in periodontal ligament proliferate under the influence of inflammation leading to formation of cystic cavity filled with pultaceous material. Most of the cysts are observed at the apex of tooth.

Microscopic Features

Cyst cavity is lined by non-keratinizing squamous epithelium penetrating underlying connective tissue. The cyst wall is composed of fibrous tissue infiltrated with mononuclear cells.

B. Developmental Cyst

1. Odontogenic Cysts

a. Dentigerous Cyst (Follicular cyst)

It arises from enamel of unerupted tooth. Usually 3rd molar of lower jaw or canine of upper jaw is involved. Commonly seen in children and young adults. It is of significance because of its reoccurrence and development of ameloblastoma and carcinoma.

Microscopic features
Cyst wall is composed of thin fibrous tissue lined by squamous epithelium.
Chronic inflammation is absent.

b. Eruption Cyst

It is cyst present over crown of unerupted tooth and is lined by squamous epithelium

c. Gingival Cyst

It arises from gingiva and lined by keratinizing squamous epithelium.

d. Primordial Cyst (Odontogenic keratocyst)

Cyst which arises from tooth forming epithelium is known as primordial cyst. Common location is 3rth molar tooth of mandible. It has tendency to recur. Cystic space is lined by keratinizing stratified squamous epithelium. Inflammatory cells are absent.

2. Nonodontogenic Cyst

a. Nasopalatine Duct Cyst

It arises from epithelial remnant of nasopalatine duct. Cyst is lined by stratified squamous epithelium or respiratory epithelium.

b. Nasolabial Cyst

Cysts present in soft tissue at nasal, maxillary process, ala of nose are derived from remnant of epithelium at nasolabial region. Cyst appears lined by squamous epithelium or respiratory epithelium.

c. Globullomaxillary Cyst

Cyst is intraosseous and is rare.

d. *Dermoid Cyst*

Cyst arises from remnant of epithelium in midline closure of mandibular and branchial arches.

ODONTOGENIC TUMORS

1. Benign

Ameloblastoma

It is a benign but locally invasive tumor. Commonly it is seen in 3rd to 5th decade of life. Tumors are located in mandibular molar area and maxilla. Tumor arises from dental epithelium of enamel, some times epithelium of dentigerous cyst or basal layer of oral mucosa.

Gross Features

Tumor is gray white, solid or cystic replacing and expanding the affected bone.

Microscopic Features

Five different patterns are seen
1. **Follicular pattern** shows follicles separated by fibrous tissue.
2. **Plexiform pattern** shows irregular plexiform masses with scanty stroma.
3. **Acanthomatous pattern** shows squamous metaplasia within the tumor masses.
4. **Basal cell pattern** shows pattern similar to basal cell carcinoma.
5. **Granular cell pattern** shows granules in the cytoplasm of tumor cells.

2. Other Benign Tumors

- **Odontogenic adenomatoid tumor:** Commonly seen on female and is associated with unerupted tooth. It shows extensive cyst formation with tubule like structures in fibrous wall of cyst.
- **Calcifying epithelial odontogenic tumor** is rare tumor exhibiting local invasiveness and recurrence. Calcific deposits are seen in stroma.
- **Odontogenic myxoma** is a locally invasive and recurring tumor. Stroma show myxomatous changes harboring odontogenic epithelium.
- **Ameloblastic fibroma** is a benign tumor occurring in younger age group. Ameloblastic epithelium is seen in very cellular connective tissue.
- **Odontomas** are hamartoma containing epithelial and mesodermal dentine tissue.
- **Cementoma** is benign tumor characterized by presence of cement or cement like substances.

3. Malignant Odontogenic Tumors

Odontogenic Carcinoma

- Malignant ameloblastoma is ameloblastoma which metastasizes.
- Ameloblastic carcinoma has cytological features of malignancy.

Odontogenic Sarcoma is rare (ameloblastic fibrosarcoma)

SALIVARY GLAND DISEASES

Salivary glands are tubuloalveolar type contain serous gland and/or mucous glands. Two groups of salivary glands are

1. Major salivary glands
   - Parotid (serous type)
   - Submandibular (mixed, predominantly serous type)
   - Sublingual (mixed, predominantly mucous type)
2. Minor salivary glands of oral mucosa (serous and/or mucous type)

Inflammatory Lesions of Salivary Glands

Sialoadenitis

Inflammation of salivary gland may be acute or chronic sialoadenitis.

Etiological Classification

1. Viral infections—Mumps, cytomegalovirus
2. Bacterial and mycotic
   A. Acute sialoadenitis: It is seen in infectious fever, postoperative and general debility conditions
   B. Chronic sialoadenitis
      - *Obstructive type:* It result from obstruction caused by calculi, trauma, surgery
      - *Non obstructive type:* Recurrent mild ascending infection from mouth cause chronic sialoadenitis
      - Chronic inflammatory diseases: Tuberculosis, actinomycosis
3. Autoimmune disease
   i. Sjögren's syndrome: It is characterized by dry eye (keratoconjunctivitis sicca), dry mouth (xerostomia) and rheumatoid arthritis.
   ii. Mikulicz's syndrome: It is characterized by sialoadenitis (inflammation of salivary gland). Inflammation of lacrimal glands and xerostomia.

Tumors of Salivary Glands

A. Benign Tumors

1. Adenoma
   a. Pleomorphic adenoma
   b. Monomorphic adenoma
2. Mesenchymal tumors

B. Malignant Tumors

1. Mucoepidermoid carcinoma
2. Malignant mixed tumors
3. Adenoid cystic carcinoma

4. Acinic cell tumor
5. Adenocarcinoma
6. Epidermoid carcinoma
7. Undifferentiated carcinoma
8. Miscellaneous

Pleomorphic Salivary Adenoma (Mixed salivary tumor)

- It is most common painless, single, slow growing tumor of major or minor salivary glands and commonest tumor of parotid gland.
- Age incidence—frequent in 3rd to 5th decades of life, more common in female.

Gross Features

- Circumscribed, pseudocapsulated, round to multilobated, firm mass
- Cut section reveals gray white to bluish semilucent, mucoid appearance

Microscopic Features (Fig. 20.4)

- Epithelial elements are mixed with mucoid, myxoid and chondroid stromal tissue
- Epithelial component form ducts, acini, tubules, sheets and strands composed of cuboidal or columnar epithelium and spindle-shaped myoepithelial cells
- Mesenchymal component is composed of loose connective tissue like mucoid, myxoid or chondroid matrix
- Homogeneous material is seen in ducts is epithelial mucin (PAS +ve) while present in stroma is connective tissue mucin (PAS -ve)

Prognosis

Recurrence is common after removal of the mass.

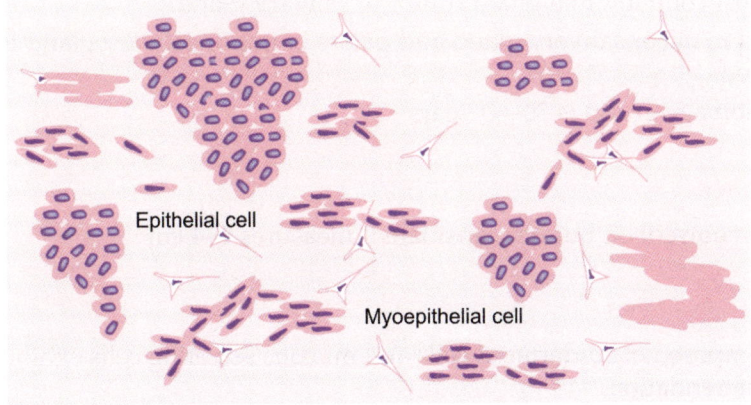

Fig. 20.4: Pleomorphic salivary adenoma

Monomorphic Adenoma

These are benign epithelial tumors without mesenchymal element.

1. Warthin's Tumor (Papillary cystadenoma lymphomatosum)

It is a benign tumor commonly seen in men in 4th to 7th decade of life.

Gross Features

- Encapsulated round or oval with smooth surface
- Cut section shows slitlike cystic space containing milky fluid and papillary projections

Microscopic Features

Tumor shows two components
1. Epithelial element is composed of glands and cystic spaces are lined by epithelium
2. Lymphoid elements are present below epithelium and may show germinal centers

2. Oxyphil Adenoma (Oncocytoma)

It is a rare slow growing benign tumor, composed of sheets, tubules and acini of large oncocytes. It is seen commonly in the 55–70 age group.

3. Others are monomorphic myoepithelioma, basal cell adenoma, and clear cell adenoma, papillary cystadenoma, and sialoadenoma papilliferum.

Malignant Salivary Gland Tumors

1. Mucoepidermoid carcinoma
   - It is most common malignant tumor of salivary gland.
   - Parotid in major salivary gland and palate in minor salivary gland is commonly involved.
   - Common age group is 30–60 years

Gross Features

Tumor is circumscribed but not capsulated, measures 1–4 cm

Microscopic Features

Tumor is composed of epidermoid cells and mucous secreting cells exhibiting various levels of differentiation.

2. Malignant mixed tumor

 Three patterns can be seen

 a. **Carcinomas arising in benign mixed salivary tumor** (common)

  Transformation occurs in later ages.

  Focal areas show features of malignancy in mixed salivary pattern.

 b. **Carcinosarcoma** (rare)

 c. **Metastasizing mixed salivary tumor** (rare)

3. Adenoid cystic carcinoma

 Highly malignant tumor, infiltrate along nerve sheath. It shows cribriform pattern of epithelial and myoepithelial cells.

4. Acinic cell carcinoma: Rare tumor, composed of sheets of acinic cells, resembling serous gland cells.

5. Adenocarcinoma and epidermoid carcinoma are similar to other parts of body and are rarely seen.

21 *Diseases of Cardiovascular System*

HEART FAILURE

Heart failure is defined as impairment of cardiac function so that heart is not able to maintain adequate circulation of blood to meet the metabolic needs of the body. Cardiac output depends upon (Fig. 21.1)

A. Preload, i.e. volume and pressure of blood in ventricles before systolic contraction of heart

B. After load, i.e. systemic peripheral resistance or pulmonary circulation resistance.

C. Strength of myocardial muscle.

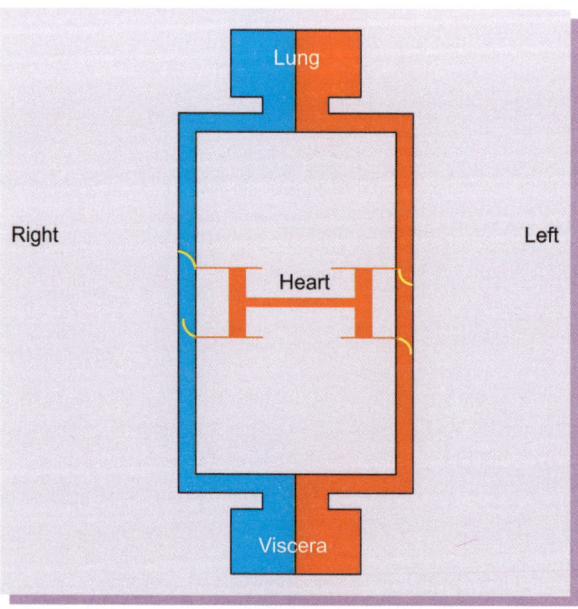

Fig. 21.1: Cardiovascular system

Classification

A. Systolic and Diastolic Heart Failure

- Systolic heart failure is because of abnormality in myocardial contraction
- Diastolic heart failure is because of abnormality in myocardial relaxation which results in poor ventricular filling

B. Acute and Chronic Heart Failure

- Rapid and sudden reduction in cardiac output occurs because of acute myocardial infarction, cardiac rupture, and massive pulmonary embolism. It results in systemic hypotension without edema (cardiogenic shock).
- Chronic heart failure develops slowly. It is seen in myocardial ischaemia, valvular disease, systemic hypertension, chronic lung diseases. In chronic heart failure compensatory mechanism try to maintain adequate cardiac output and edema develops.

C. Left Sided and Right Sided Heart Failure

Left functional unit of heart undergo failure because of systemic hypertension, mitral/aortic valve disease, ischaemic heart disease, cardiomyopathy. Clinical manifestations results from

- Increased left atrial pressure transmitted to lung leading to pulmonary congestion.
- Decreased left ventricular output leading to hypoxic and ischaemic changes in kidney, brain, and skeletal muscles (Fig. 21.2).

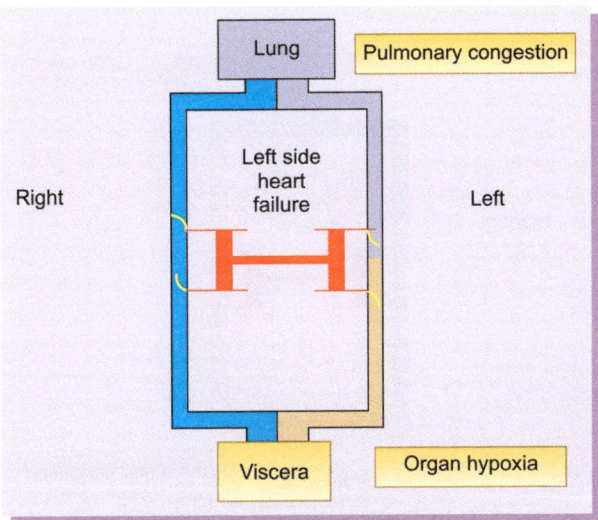

Fig. 21.2: Left side heart failure

- Right sided heart failure occurs because of intrinsic lung disease (cor pulmonale), pulmonary valve disease, and pulmonary hypertension or as a consequence of left ventricular failure (Fig. 21.3).

Clinical Manifestations Results From

- Systemic and portal venous congestion leading to edema, congestion of liver, spleen, kidney, ascitis, pleural effusion, congested neck, and leg veins.
- Reduced cardiac output leads to anoxia and cyanosis.

D. Forward and Backward Heart Failure

Forward Heart Failure

Clinical manifestations are because of diminished blood flow to the tissue, especially decreased renal perfusion leading to activation of rennin-angiotensin mechanism.

Backward Heart Failure

Increased volume and pressure in atrium is transmitted back leading to venous congestion in lungs and tissues.

E. High Output and Low Output Failure

- High output failure is associated with increased output. For example, hyperthyroidism, anaemia, pregnancy, A-V fistula and beriberi.
- Low output is associated with low cardiac output. For example, ischaemic heart disease, hypertension, valvular diseases, and pericardial disease.

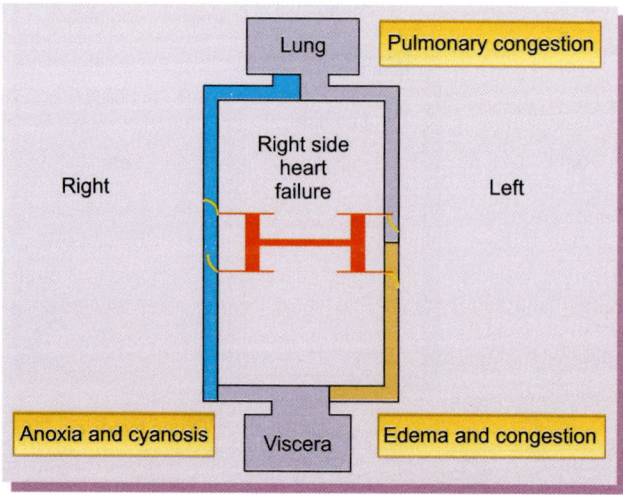

Fig. 21.3: Right side heart failure

Etiology

I. *Intrinsic Pump Failure*

- Ischaemic heart disease
- Myocarditis
- Cardiomyopathy
- Cardiac conduction disorders

II. *Increased Workload*

- Systemic and pulmonary hypertension
- Aortic and pulmonary valvular diseases (stenosis)
- Chronic pulmonary diseases
- High output failure

III. *Impaired Filling*

- Mitral and tricuspid stenosis
- Cardiac temponade, pericarditis

Clinical Manifestations

1. Dyspnoea: Initially on exertion later on at rest
2. Orthopnoea: Dyspnoea in recumbent position (lying flat)
3. Paroxysmal nocturnal dyspnoea: Dyspnoea at night
4. Cyanosis: Bluish coloration of mucosa and nail bed
5. Tachycardia, hypotension, engorged neck vein
6. Congestive hepatomegaly
7. Pleural, peritoneal and pericardial effusion
8. Pulmonary edema and edema feet
9. Nonspecific symptoms like anorexia, nausea, pain abdomen, weakness, low-grade fever

Diagnosis

- X-ray chest shows cardiomegaly
- ECG shows arrhythmia, ischaemic changes
- Echocardiography

CONGENITAL HEART DISEASE

These are present since birth and accounts for 0.5% of newborn children. It is attributed to multifactorial inheritance involving genetic and environmental factors, like rubella, drugs, alcohol, etc.

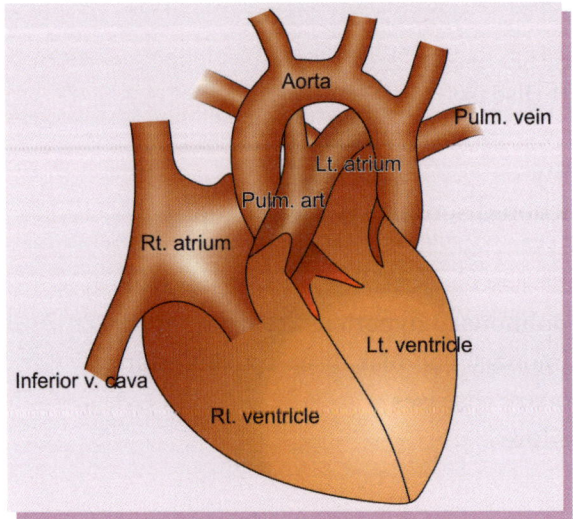

Fig. 21.4: Normal heart

Classification

A. *Malposition of Heart like Dextrocardia* (Right side placement of heart)

B. *Shunts*

   1. Left to right
- Ventricular septal defect (VSD)
- Atrial septal defect (ASD)
- Patent ductus arteriosus (PDA)

   2. Right to left
- Tetralogy of Fallot (TOF)
- Transposition of great arteries
- Persistent trunchus arteriosus
- Tricuspid atresia and stenosis

C. *Obstruction*

   i. Coarctation of aorta

  ii. Aortic stenosis and atresia

 iii. Pulmonary stenosis and atresia

1. *Left to Right Shunt* (Acyanotic group or late cyanotic)

There is shunting of blood from left side to right side of heart resulting in volume overload on right heart, producing pulmonary hypertension and right ventricular hypertrophy. At later stage, pressure on right side is higher than left side resulting in cyanotic heart disease.

Ventricular Septal Defect (VSD)

There is a gap between right and left ventricles. It is most common heart disease (30%). Small defect closes spontaneously and larger defect produce significant effect (Fig. 21.5).

Types
- Most commonly located type is close to the bundle of His, involving membranous septum (90% cases)
- Rest 10% involves muscular septum placed below pulmonary or aortic valve

Effects
- Right ventricular hypertrophy, right atrial hypertrophy
- Enlargement and haemodynamic changes in tricuspid and pulmonary valves
- Left ventricular and atrial volume hypertrophy
- Enlargement and haemodynamic changes in mitral and aortic valves

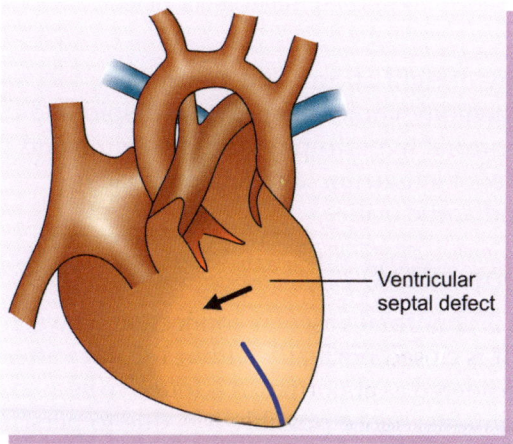

Ventricular septal defect

Fig. 21.5: Ventricular septal defect

Atrial Septal Defect (ASD)

There is a gap betweent two atria. It comprises of 10% of congenital heart disease and remains unnoticed in childhood till pulmonary hypertension cause late cyanotic heart disease (Fig. 21.6).

Types
- In 90% cases it is present in the region of fossa ovalis (osteum secondum type)
- In 5% cases defect lies low in inter atrial septum, adjacent to A-V valve. It may be associated with aortic/mitral valve defect producing insufficiency (osteum primum type)
- In rest 5% cases defect is located high in inter atrial septum near entry of superior vena cava (sinus venosus type)

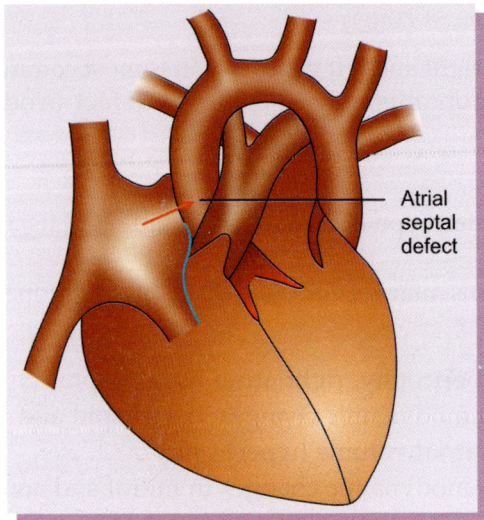

Fig. 21.6: Atrial septal defect

Effects
- Volume hypertrophy of right atrium and ventricle
- Enlargement and haemodynamic changes in tricuspid and pulmonary valves
- Focal/diffuse endocardial hypertrophy of right atrium and ventricles
- Volume hypertrophy of left atrium and left ventricle
- Small size mitral and aortic orifice

Patent Ductus Arteriosus (PDA)

The ductus arteriosus is abnormal vascular connection between aorta and bifurcation of pulmonary artery. It is closed normally within 1–2 days after delivery. If it persists after 3 months, it is considered as abnormal. It is found to be associated with respiratory distress syndrome in infants; hence possibly it is due to persistent synthesis of PGE_2 after birth. PDA may be 2 cm in length and 1 cm in diameter (Fig. 21.7).

Effects
- Volume hypertrophy of left atrium and ventricle
- Enlargement and haemodynamic changes in mitral and pulmonary valve
- Enlargement of ascending aorta

2. Right to Left Shunt (Cyanotic heart disease)

Poorly oxygenated blood in systemic circulation results in early cyanosis.

Tetralogy of Fallot (Fig. 21.8)

It is most common cyanotic congenital heart disease. Characteristic features are:
A. VSD
B. Overriding of aorta

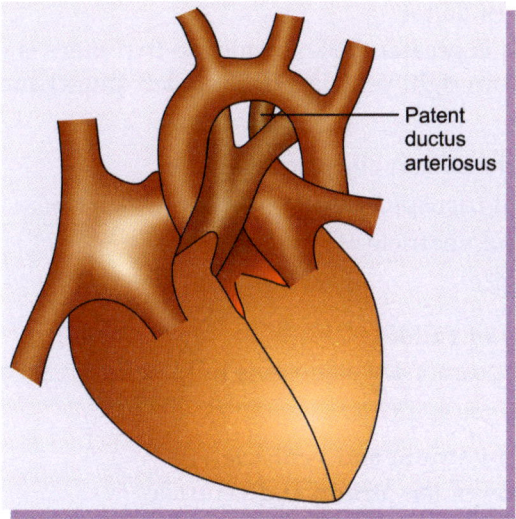

Fig. 21.7: Patent ductus arteriosus

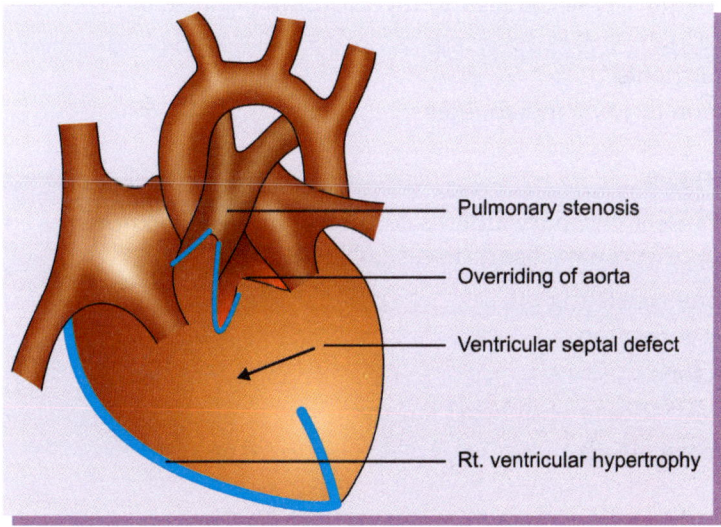

Fig. 21.8: Tetralogy of Fallot

C. Pulmonary stenosis
D. Right ventricular hypertrophy

Depending on severity of the disease extent of pulmonary stenosis and size of VSD it is of two types.

A. Cyanotic tetralogy of Fallot

Pulmonary stenosis is greater. VSD is mild, so that there is more resistance to the outflow of blood from right ventricle (right to left shunt) and cyanosis.

Effects are
- Hypertrophy of right atrium and ventricle
- Small and abnormal tricuspid valve
- Small left atrium and ventricle
- Enlarged aortic orifice

B. Acyanotic tetralogy of Fallot

VSD is greater and pulmonary stenosis is mild (left to right shunt)

Effects are
- Hypertrophy of right atrium and ventricle
- Volume hypertrophy of left atrium and ventricle
- Enlargement of mitral and aortic orifice

ISCHAEMIC HEART DISEASE

Diseases which results from myocardial ischaemia are known as ischaemic heart diseases. Ischaemia cause damage to myocardium because of
- Hypoxia
- Deficient nutrients
- Accumulation of toxic metabolites

Etiopathogenesis

Commonest cause is coronary atherosclerosis therefore also known as coronary artery disease (CAD) or coronary heart disease (CHD).

It is a syndrome consisting of:
- Myocardial infarction
- Angina pectoris
- Chronic heart disease with heart failure
- Sudden cardiac death

Syndrome is as the result of interaction between (Fig. 21.9)
A. Fixed atherosclerotic narrowing
B. Thrombosis over disrupted plaque (acute plaque changes)
C. Platelet aggregation and vasospasm

A. Fixed Coronary Narrowing

- At least >75% reduction of cross sectional area in one coronary artery, and usually 2–3 arteries are involved by atherosclerosis.

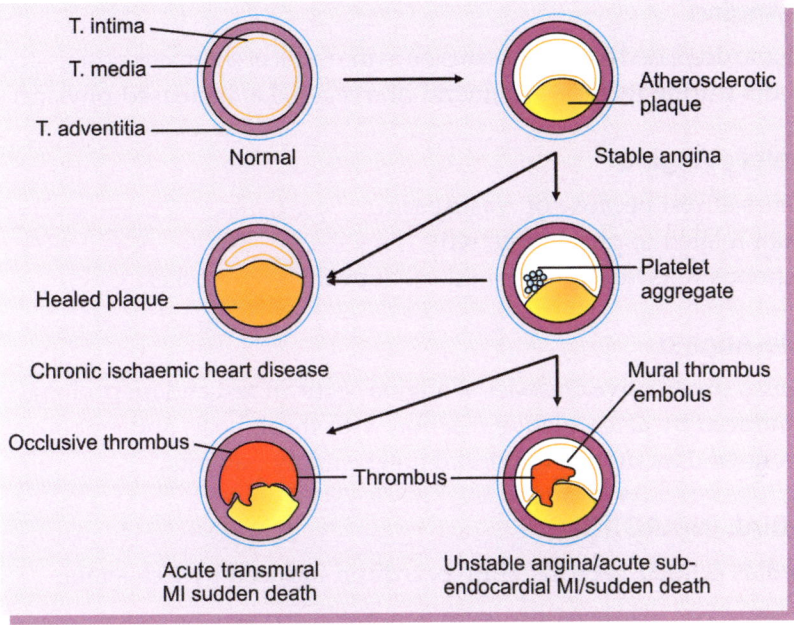

Fig. 21.9: Coronary artery disease

- Order of involvement is left anterior descending, left circumflex artery, right coronary artery producing clinically significant changes.
- Intramural branches are not atherosclerosed.

B. *Acute Plaque Changes*

- Exposure of thrombogenic surface to blood leads to thrombus formation over disrupted plaque.
- Other contributory factors affecting acute plaque changes are:
  - Adrenergic stimulation
  - Eccentric plaque
  - Rate and degree of obstruction.

C. *Platelet Aggregation and Vasospasm*

It is responsible for Prinzmetal's angina and acute myocardial infarction.

ANGINA PECTORIS

It is paroxysmal recurrent substernal/precordial chest discomfort caused by transient ischaemia (15 sec. to 15 mts), which falls short for induction of cellular necrosis, i.e. infarction. Three patterns of angina pectoris are

1. Stable angina
2. Prinzmetal's angina
3. Unstable angina

1. Stable Angina

- It is due to decreased coronary perfusion as the result of chronic stenosing atherosclerosis.
- It occurs during increased demand of oxygen, i.e. increased physical exercise.

2. Prinzmetal's Angina

- It occurs at rest because of vasospasm.
- It is not related to physical activity.
- It responds to nitroglycerine and calcium channel blocker.

3. Unstable Angina

- Repeated progressive episodes of angina occur, at rest and for prolonged duration.
- It is induced by acute plaque reaction with thrombosis and embolization.
- It is followed by myocardial infarction in many patients.

MYOCARDIAL INFARCTION

It is defined as cellular necrosis of myocardium induced by ischaemia.

Risk Factors

- Risk of myocardial infarction increases with age
- More common in male as compared to female
- Risk is increased with hypertension, diabetes mellitus, hyperlipidaemia, increased homocysteine level
- Severe coronary atherosclerosis and acute plaque reaction leads to thrombosis and acute myocardial infarction

Pathogenesis

Ischaemia leads to biochemical changes which decrease ATP production resulting in lactic acidosis.

- If ischaemia persist for 20–40 minutes then myocardial infarction occur
- If myocardial tissue is reperfused within 15–20 minutes, then no infarction occur and thrombus is lysed or partial haemorrhagic infarction occurs.

Morphological Changes

Time lapsed	Gross features of heart	Microscopic features
0–4 hrs	No changes	Waviness of fibers at borders
4–12 hrs	No changes	Beginning of coagulative necrosis and edema
12–24 hrs	Dark mottled appearance	Coagulative necrosis, neutrophilic exudates, eosinophilia and contraction band necrosis appear

Contd...

Contd...

Time lapsed	Gross features of heart	Microscopic features
1–3 days	Hyperaemia around yellow infarced center	Disintegration of dead tissue followed by phagocytosis
3–7 days	Yellow tan soft with hyperaemic border	Formation of granulation tissue at border
7–10 days	Red gray depressed infarced area	Granulation tissue with fibrosis
10–14 days	Gray white scar	Increased collagen deposition
2–8 weeks	Scarred area	Dense scar tissue

Clinical Features

- Chest pain
- Rapid feeble pulse
- Dyspnoea
- Indigestion and apprehension

Consequences and Complications

- Death may occur within one hour of onset.
- If no death then, residual effects are:
  - Contractile dysfunction (left ventricular failure/cardiogenic shock
  - Arrhythmia, sinus tachycardia, bradycardia, ventricular premature beat, ventricular tachycardia, fibrillation, asystole and heart block
  - Myocardial rupture, haemopericardium, cardiac temponade, papillary muscle rupture, pseudoaneurysm.
  - Pericarditis
  - Mural thrombosis and thromboembolism
  - Ventricular aneurysm formation
  - Mitral regurgitation
  - Progressive late heart failure

Diagnosis

WHO criteria are:
- Chest pain
- ECG changes
- Increased cardiac markers like CK-MB, troponin, LDH, myoglobin estimation
- Other tests are echocardiogram, radionuclide scan, perfusion scintigraphy, MRI

INFECTIVE ENDOCARDITIS

Invasion of heart valve or endocardium by bacteria leads to infective or bacterial endocarditis.

Types

1. Acute bacterial endocarditis (ABE)
2. Subacute bacterial endocarditis (SABE)

1. Acute Endocarditis

It is characterized by destructive, necrotizing, ulcerative lesion by virulent bacteria. Usually normal valves are affected. Death occurs with in days to weeks in 50% of patients in spite of antibiotics.

2. Subacute Bacterial Endocarditis

It is characterized by less destructive lesion by less virulent organism and usually affects previously diseased heart.

Predisposing Factors

- Bacteraemia, septicemia, pyaemia
- Underlying heart disease like rheumatic heart disease, congenital heart disease
- Impaired host defense, for example in immunodeficiency, diabetes mellitus, and neutropenia.

Organisms

- *Staph aureus, Staph viridans, Staph epidermidis*
- *Haemophilus, Actinobactor, Eikenella, Cardiobacterium, Kingella* (HAECK)
- Other less common—Tuberculosis, syphilis, fungus, viral, rickettsial

Gross Features

- Mitral and aortic valves are frequently affected
- Vegetations are seen on atrial surface of A-V valve and ventricular surface of semilunar valve (Fig. 21.10).
- Acute bacterial endocarditis (ABE) vegetations are larger than subacute bacterial endocarditis (SABE)

Microscopic Features

- Outer layer of vegetation is composed of fibrin and platelet
- Middle layer shows bacterial colonies
- Deeper layer shows nonspecific inflammation

Clinical Features

Fever with chills, weakness and malaise, weight loss

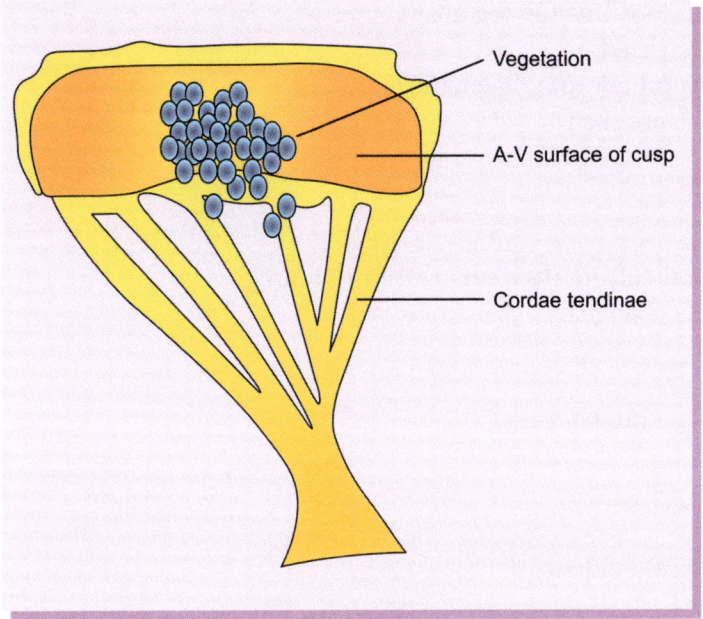

Fig. 21.10: Vegetation of infective endocarditis

Complications

A. Cardiac complications
- Valvular stenosis/regurgitation
- Perforation, rupture, aneurysm of heart
- Abscess in valve ring
- Suppurative pericarditis
- Cardiac failure

B. Extracardiac complications
  Embolism

Cause of Death

- Cardiac failure
- Renal failure
- Rupture of aneurysm

Laboratory Diagnosis

1. Blood tests
   i. Complete blood count shows leukocytosis
   ii. ESR is raised
   iii. CRP positive

2. Blood culture positive for organism
3. C3, C4 is decreased
4. Urine shows proteinuria, haematuria
5. ECG changes are seen

Diagnostic Criteria

Major

- Positive blood culture (two sets within 12 hours)
- Positive ECG changes

Minor

- Predisposing valvular lesion
- Fever
- Embolism
- Vasculitis
- Microbiological evidence
- ECG changes

To Diagnose Endocarditis

- Two major criteria
- One major and 3 minor criteria
- Five minor criteria

ATHEROSCLEROSIS

It is characterized by deposition of fibro-fatty plaque in the intima of large- and medium-sized muscular arteries.

Risk Factors

A. Major Risk Factors

Constitutional Risk Factors

- Atherosclerosis increases with age
- Males are more at risk than females
- More risk in hereditary derangement of lipoprotein
- Familial clusters of hypertension are at more risk atherosclerosis
- Diabetes mellitus patients are at more risk of atherosclerosis

Acquired Risk Factors

- Hyperlipidaemia
- High cholesterol level

- Hypertension
- Diabetes mellitus
- Smoking

B. *Minor Risk Factors*

- Environmental
- Sedentary lifestyle of people
- Type A personality
- Obesity
- Lack of exercise
- Homocystinuria
- Infections (*Chlamydia*, Herpes has been found in coronary plaque)
- Alcohol is beneficial by raising HDL cholesterol

Pathogenesis

Reaction to Injury Theory

- Injury to endocardium due to risk factors cause platelet aggregation
- Infiltration of monocytes and lymphocytes in vessel wall
- Release of cytokines induce smooth muscle proliferation
- LDL is oxidized by free radicals; oxidized LDL is ingested by macrophages and formation of fatty streaks occur
- Endothelial disruption by fatty streaks leads to further aggregation of platelets
- Smooth muscle proliferation leads to fibrous plaque formation (Fig. 21.11)
- Fibrous plaque undergo dystrophic calcification, haemorrhage, thrombosis and ulceration to form complicated atheromatous plaque (Fig. 21.12).

Morphological Features

1. *Fatty Streaks*

These are precursor of atheroma, but are harmless. These are multiple flat or elevated linear yellow spots 1 mm to 1 cm in length, composed of foam cells, lipid containing smooth muscle cells and T lymphocytes.

2. *Gelatinous Lesions*

These are round to oval gray elevations, composed of increased ground substance in intima.

3. *Atheromatous Plaque*

These are yellow white 1–2 cm in size raised above surface, composed of yellow grumous lipid covered by white fibrous cap.

Clinical Features and Complications

1. Myocardial infarction

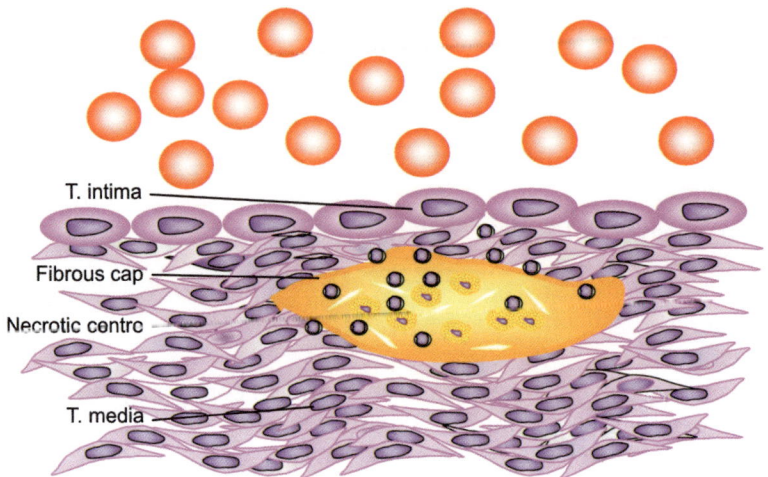

Fig. 21.11: Morphological changes in atherosclerosis

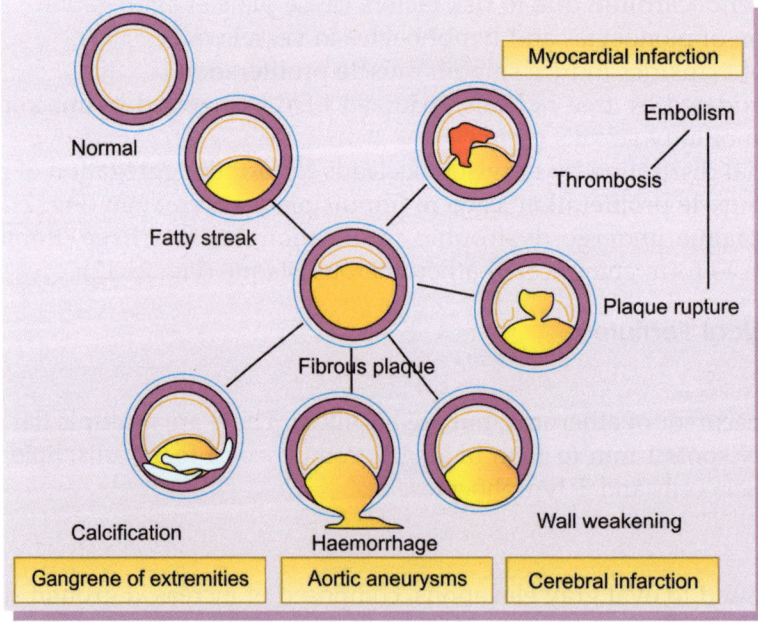

Fig. 21.12: Progression and complications of atherosclerosis

2. Cerebral stroke
3. Calcification, ulceration, thrombosis, haemorrhage and aneurysm
4. Intermittent claudication and peripheral vascular disease
5. Embolization
6. Ischaemic infarction of bowel
7. Reno-vascular hypertension

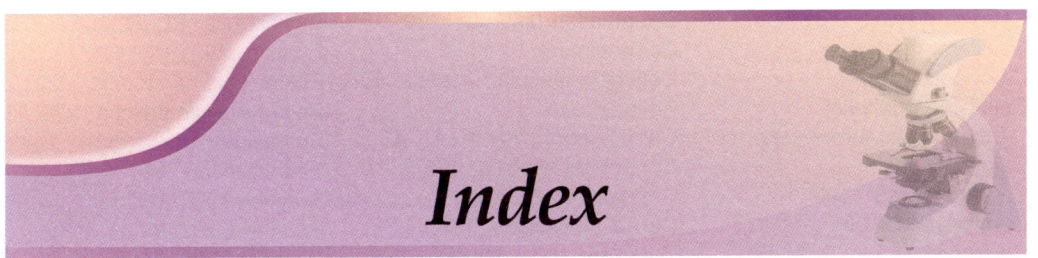

Index